The Disea[...]

INFANTS & CHILDREN

and their

Homoeopathic and General Treatment

with

Glossory and Therapeutic Index

E. HARRIS RUDDOCK, M.D.

Licentiate of the Royal College of Member of the
Royal College of Surgeons; Licentiath in Midwifery
(London and Edinburgh), etc.; Late Physician to
Reading and Berkshire Homoeopathic dispensary

EIGHTH EDITION, REVISED AND LARGELY RE-WRITTEN
by
T. MILLER NEATBY
M.A., M.D. (CANTAB) ; M.A. (LOND.)

B. JAIN PUBLISHERS (P) LTD.

INFANTS & CHILDREN
and their
Homoeopathic and General Treatment

Price: Rs. 65.00

Published by **Kuldeep Jain**

for **B. Jain Publishers (P) Ltd.**
1921, Street No. 10, Chuna Mandi,
Paharganj, New Delhi–110 055 (INDIA)
Phones: 91-011-2358 0800, 2358 1100, 2358 1300
Fax: 91-011-2358 0471; Email: bjain@vsnl.com
Website: www.bjainbooks.com

Printed in India by
J. J. Offset Printers
522, FIE, Patpar Ganj, Delhi–110 092
Phones: 91-011-2216 9633, 2215 6128
ISBN: 81-7021-313-4
BOOK CODE: BR-2454

Preface to the
EIGHTH EDITION

A NEW edition of Ruddock's *Diseases of Infants and Children* having been impreatively called for, it was decided to overhaul thoroughly this popular work and to bring it, especially with regard to its pathology and its non-medical treatment, up to present date. This has involved a good deal of re-writing and the addition of several supplementary sections, notably sections on Tonsils and Adenoids, Rheumatism in Children, Appendicitis and Bacilluria. Some hints on the place of operation in such affections as tonsils and adenoids, appendicitis, etc., have, it is believed, both widened the outlook of the book and added to its value. The action and value of homoeopathic medication remains the same from generation to generation, and little alteration has been made in the parts of the work that deal with this subject. In spite of necessary alterations and additions, the general plan and arrangement of the book has been studiously preserved.

T. MILLER NEARBY
102 RIGGINDALE ROAD,
STREATHAM.

Preface to the
FIRST EDITION

AFTER LONG but unavoidable delay this Manual on children's diseases in sent forth on its errand. It makes no pretensions to be an exhaustive treatise, to write which the author has not had sufficient time at this disposal; it is simply a practical contribution to the alleviation and cure of those diseases which are of most frequent and fatal occurrence. The book is intended to be a companion-volume to *The Lady's Manual of Homoeopathic Treatment*. Taken together, they deal with subjects of the highest importance to individuals, to families, and to the community at large. From healthy mothers and a healthy progeny—sound in mind and body—we may expect future generations of healthy men and women.

The present work is, from beginning to end, based on *preventive* as well as curative treatment. The author, having great faith in the principles and practice enunciated, anticipates the best results from its publication, whenever its hygienic and medical prescriptions are fairly adopted and persistently carried out.

In the treatment of children there is much to encourage the practitioner. Their diseases are generally uncomplicated by internal organic changes, and by those deep and complex disorders of nutrition which result from the abused organs or over-used brains of the middle-aged, or of those degenerative changes which are to be found in the body during the decline of life. Neither are children liable to that emotional *depression* which often tells so disastrously on the recovery of adults. With them memory has nothing regretful to recall, and, after an illness, hope rises with exultant wing. They live emphatically in the present, and are exempt from the despondency which, in mature life, is apt to attend reflections on the *past* or anticipation of the *future*.

Sometimes, however, the desired victory is not gained : disease triumphs, and a young life is lost, leaving a blank in the domestic circle which cannot soon be filled. The silence that regins in the house, the vacant nursery, the unused toys, the treasured clothing, all speak eloquently and mournfully of the loss which is sustained by the bereaved household, and which frequently awakens the deep symptahy of the physician whose skill and care have been frustrated. Happily, the reverse of this generally happens, and the agony of suspense—so exquisitely expressed by David, "Who can tell whether God will be gractious unto me, that the child may live ?" —is relieved, and the child,just now so seriously ill, recovers, to make his parents happy, perhaps to accomplish a great work, and to leave a name in which posterity will rejoice.

The book is not simply a combination from other works of the author. Some of the sections are entirely new; and in all of them important additions and alterations have been made, so as to bring the work abreast with the most recent advances in medicine; while such special points on diagnosis and treatment have been introduced as are calculated to render the Manual a useful guide to the treatment of the diseases of infancy and childhood.

The author has much pleasure in acknowledging his indebtedness to Dr. Lade for very effective help. He has read over a large portion of the work in manuscript, and added some valuable notes, which will be found in various parts of the Manual. It is sent forth with the earnest hope that it may prove a boon to many little ones.

E. H. RUDDOCK

Preface to the
FIFTH EDITION

IN THE edition of this Manual, first published after the lamented death of Dr. Ruddock, some alterations and additions were made by Dr. Lade, who had rendered considerable help to the author in the original preparation of the work ; most of the notes with his initials G.L. appended have been retained. For the present edition the publishers are indebted to Dr. John H. Charke, Physician to the London Homoeopathic Hospital, who has endevoured to bring the work fully abreast with the times. The whole of the Manual has been carefully revised, numerous additions made, and new improvements in treatment have been taken account of. A new section on German Measles has been added ; and a Appendix calling attention to the necesity in some cases of commencing the treatment of children before their birth. The Glossary has been enlarged ; and every care taken to make the work as practical and available as possible. It is hoped that the new edition will prove in every way worthy of the preceding ones, which have already met with such a hearty reception from the public.

Note on the
SIXTH AND SEVENTH EDITIONS

IN PRESENTING a new edition of this Manual, the publishers have thought it inadvisable to make any radical alteration. The work has been carefully read and corrections made where necessary, but in all its essentials the book will be found identical with its immediate predecessor.

12 WARWICK LANE,
LONDON.

Contents

PART (I)
Introductory

Chapter I
The Medicines

Medicines recommended for children—List
of remedies recommended for infants and
children—Directions respecting the medicines.

Chapter II
General Directions for the Management of Infants

The new-born infant—Still-born infants—
Washing and bathing—The warm bath—
Clothing—Sleep—Open-air exercise.

Chapter III
Examples of Dietary for Healthy Children, at Different Ages

For the first six months—Diet from nine

PART (II)

Diseases of Infants and Children, and their Homoeopathic and General Treatment

Chapter I
Acute Specific Diseases

Scarlet fever, scarlatina—Post-Scarlatinal dropsy—Measles—German measles—Small-pox—Vaccination, Cow-pox—Chicken- pox—Simple fever—Enteric fever, Typhoid fever—Diphtheria—Whooping-cough—Mumps.

Chapter II
Constitutional Diseases

Rheumatism of children—Rickets—Tuber-culous diseases of bones and glands—Tubercular meningitis—Consumption of the bowels—Muco-purulent ophthalmia.

Chapter III
Diseases of the Nervous System

Chronic hydrocephalus, Water on the brain—Infantile convulsions, fits—Spasmodic croup, Child-crowing—Epilepsy, Falling-sickness—Infantile paralysis—Chorea, St. Vitus's dance—Headache—Sleeplessness.

Chapter IV
Diseases of the Eye, Ear, etc.

Purulent Inflammation of the eyes

of the spine, skoliosis—Swelling of infants'
breasts—Ruptured navel—Incontinence of
urine, Wetting the bed—Bacilluria.

Chapter I

THE MEDICINES

MEDICINES RECOMMENDED FOR CHILDREN

A Chest containing the necessary homoeopathic medicines for the treatment of infantile diseases should be always kept in readiness in every house in which there are children. The importance of this recommendation will be fully apparent when the peculiarities of the organism of the little patients are considered.

In consequence of the activity of the vital powers, and the quickness and force of the circulation, there is a remarkable susceptibility to inflammatory action in children, so that many of their diseases rapidly run on to organic and incurable mischief. **Active Circulation**

The earliest recognition of an approaching illness, and the most prompt application of treatment, are therefore of the greatest importance. Neglect or delay may prove most disastrous to life, while a few doses of an appropriate remedy timely administered will often be alone sufficient to arrest the morbid process, or they will afford temporary relief till the arrival of a physician. **Prompt Administration**

In the treatment of infants, perseverance and watchfulness

and necessary. Patient attention should be given to the investigation of every ailment, and no case should ever be abandoned as altogether hopeless. It is well known that children often recover from the most severe diseases, and, in the great majority of instances, especially if taken in time, the balance will quickly turn in the right direction. **Perseverance**

The absence of nauseousness from homoeopathic medicines is an advantage which mothers can appreciate who have witnessed the natural and proper disgust of children to draughts and pills. The agreeableness of the remedies is, however, only a minor advantage of the treatment.

The medicines used in homoeopathic practice are prepared in different forms—*Globules, Pilules, Tinctures,* and *Triturations.* Globules are now almost wholly superseded by Pilules ; and Triturations are seldom used except in profess-ional practice. A description of the different forms may be found in *The Stepping-stone to Homoeopathy and Health,* pp. 63, 65 (210th thousand) ; and in the *Vade Mecum of Modern Medi-cine Surgery* (115th thousand).   **Forms of Medicines**

LIST OF REMEDIES RECOMMENDED FOR INFANTS AND CHILDREN

Name	Abbreviation	Attenuation
1. Acidum Hydrocyanicum	ACID.-HYDROCY.	3x
2. Acidum Muriaticum	ACID.-MUR.	3x
3. Acidum Phosphoricum	ACID.-PHOS	3x
4. Aconitum Napellus	ACON.	3x
5. Agaricus Muscatius	AGAR.	3x
6. Ailanthus Glandulosa	AILANTH.	1
7. Ammonium Carbonicum	AMMON.-CARB.	1
8. Antimonium Tartaricum	ANT.-TART.	3x
9. Antimonium Crudum	ANT.-CRUD.	3x
10. Apis Mellifica	APIS.	3x

11. Aralia	ARAL.	3x
12. Argentum Nitricum	ARG.-NIT.	4
13. Arnica Montana	ARN.	3x
14. Arsenicum Album	ARS.	3x
15. Arsenicum Iodidum	ARS.-IOD.	3x
16. Aurum Metallicum	AUR.-MET.	5
17. Baptisia Tinctoria	BAPT.	1x
18. Belladonna	BELL.	3x
19. Bromium	BROM.	1
20. Bryonia Alba	BRY.	3x
21. Calcarea Carbonica	CALC.-C.	5
22. Calcarea Phosphorata	CALC.-P.	3x
23. Cantharis Vesicatoria	CANTH.	3x
24. Carbo Vegetabilis	CARBO. V.	5
25. Chamomilla Matricaria	CHAM.	3
26. China Officinalis	CHIN.	3x
27. Cina Anthelmintica	CIN.	3x
28. Coffea Cruda	COFF.	3x
29. Colocynthis	COLOC.	3x
30. Croton Tiglium	CROT-T.	6
31. Cuprum Metallicum	CUP.-M.	5
32. Curare	CURARE.	3
33. Drosera Rotundifolia	DROS.	3x
34. Dulcamara	DULC.	3x
35. Euphrasia Officinalis	EUPH.	1
36. Ferrum Iodidum	FERR.-I.	3x
37. Gelseminum Sempervirens	GELS.	3x
38. Glonoine	GLON.	3x
39. Graphites	GRAPH.	5
40. Guaiacum	GUAIA.	1
41. Hamamelis Virginica	HAM.	1
42. Helleborus Niger	HELL.	3x
43. Hepar Sulphuris Calcareum	HEP.-S.	3x
44. Hyoscyamus Niger	HYOS.	3x
45. Ignatia Amara	IGN.	3x
46. Iodium	IOD.	3x
47. Ipecacuanha	IPEC.	3x
48. Iris Versicolor	IRIS.	1
49. Kali Hydriodicum	K.-HYD.	3x
50. Kreasotum	KREOS.	3x

51. Lathyrus Statious	LATH.-S.	3
52. Mercurius Biniodatus	MERC.-BIN.	3x
53. Mercurius Iodatus	MERC.-IOD.	2x
54. Mercurius Corrosivus	MERC.-COR.	3x
55. Mercurius Cyanatus	MERC.-CYAN.	6
56. Mercurius Solubilis	MERC.-SOL.	3x and 6 x
57. Nux Vomica	NUX.-V.	3x
58. Opium	OPI.	3x
59. Phosphorus	PHOS.	3
60. Plantago	PLANT.	3
61. PodophyllumPeltatum	PODOPH.	1x
62. Pulsatilla Nigricans	PULS.	3x
63. Plumbum Aceticum	PLUMB.-AC.	3
64. Rhus Toxicodendron	RHUS.	3x
65. Rheum	RHEUM.	1
66. Silicea	SIL.	6
67. Spongia Tosta	SPONG.	3x
68. Stramonium	STRAM.	3
69. Staphysagria	STAPH.	3x
70. Sulphur	SULPH.	3
71. Veratrum Album	VERAT.-A.	3x
72. Veratrum Viride	VERAT.-V.	3x
73. Zincum	ZINC.	5

Camphor (Rubini's Tincture, or Camphor Pilules) should also be procured, but kept separate from the rest.

External Remedies—The following remedies, in strong tinctures, will be found invaluable for the accidents to which children are liable :—

Arnica, Calendula, Cantharis, and Rhus Toxicodendron.

THE TWENTY-FOUR CHIEF REMEDIES

Name	Abbreviation	Attenuation
1. Aconitum Napellus	ACON.	3x
2. Arnica Montana	ARN.	3x

3.	Arsenicum Album	ARS.	3x
4.	Belladonna	BELL.	3x
5.	Bryonia	BRY.	3x
6.	Calcarea Carbonica	CALC.-C	5
7.	Calcarea Phosphorata	CALC.-P.	3x
8.	Chamomilla Matricaria	CHAM.	3x
9.	China Officinalis	CHIN.	3x
10.	Cina Anthelmintica	CIN.	3x
11.	Coffea Cruda	COFF.	3x
12.	Drosera Rotundifolia	DROS.	3x
13.	Gelseminum Sempervirens	GELS.	3x
14.	Hepar Sulphuris Calcareum	HEP.-S.	3x
15.	Ipecacuanha	IPEC.	3x
16.	Mercurius Solubilus	MERC.-SOL.	6
17.	Nux Vomica	NUX.-V.	3
18.	Phosphorus	PHOS.	3
19.	Pulstilla Nigricans	PULS.	3x
20.	Rhus Toxicodendron	RHUS.	3x
21.	Silicea	SIL.	6
22.	Spongia Tosta	SPONG.	3x
23.	Sulphur	SULPH.	3x
24.	Veratrum Album	VERAT.-V.	3x

If the foregoing remedies are kept in Pilules or Globules the attenuation of some of them must be slightly modified, according to the discretion of a qualified homoeopathic chemist.

DIRECTIONS RESPECTING THE MEDICINES

Pilules or globules may be taken dry on the tongue, but it is better, when convenient, to dissolve them in pure soft water.

If tinctures are used, a little practice is necessary to drop them with accuracy. Before removing the cork, invert the bottle so as to wet the end of the cork. The required quantity should be dropped into the bottom of a glass by holding the bottle in an oblique manner, with the lip resting against the middle of the end of the cork (see illustration), when the tincture will descend and drop from the lower edge of the cork; or a piece of solid glass, about 1/16 of an inch diameter,

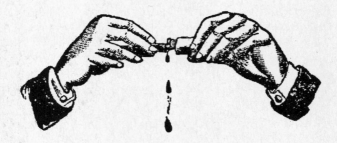

bent at a right angle, and introduced into the bottle, will so enable the most timid to drop the tinctures with exactness.*

Water, in the proportion of a dessert-spoonful to a drop,

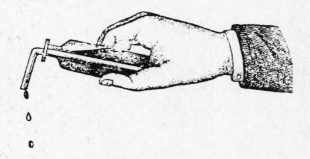

should then be poured upon the medicine. For infants who object to cold water, the spoon may be warmed by dipping it in hot water, and then the medicine added to about half a teaspoonful of water. The vessel should be scrupulously

---

* Drop conductors for the above purpose can be obtained from the Homoeopathic chemists.

clean, and, if the mixture has to stand some time after being made, it should be covered over with a saucer or sheet of notepaper. The spoon should be always wiped after being used. and put away in a clean place till again required. Fine glazed earthenware or glass spoons are the best for this purpose. If the medicine has to be kept several days, cold boiled water should be employed, and the mixture put into a *new* bottle, particular care being taken that the cork is new and sound. To protect the medicines from light and dust, and to distinguish them from other liquids graduated earthenware medicine-cups, with covers, specially made for this purpose, are the best, and may be procured of any homoeopathic chemist.

Hours—The most appropriate times for administering the medicines, as a rule, are—on rising in the morning, at bedtime, and, if oftener prescribed, about and hour before or after a meal.

The Dose—In determining the quantity and strength of doses, several circumstances require consideration, such as age, sex, habits, nature of the disease, organ involved, and the susceptibility to the medicine. As before stated, the circulation of children is quicker than that of adults, and the nervous system more impressible ; the dose has therefore to be regulated by these peculiarities.

With the above exceptions, and allowing for any peculiarity of constitution, the following general directions may be given as to the dose :—

One drop of Tincture or two Pilules. For young infants, one half or one third of the above quantities.

A Pilule, or one drop, is easily divided into two or more does, by mixing it with two or more spoonfuls of water, and giving one spoonful for a dose.

Repetition of Doses—In this matter we must be guided by the acute or chronic character of the malady, the urgency and danger of the symptoms, and the effects produced by the medicines. In violent and acute diseases, such as Croup, Convulsions, etc., the remedies may be repeated every fifteen, twenty, or thirty minutes ; in less urgent cases, every two, three, or four hours. In chronic maladies the medicine may be administered every six, twelve, or twenty-four hours. In all cases when improvement takes place, the medicine should be taken less frequently, and gradually relinquished.

Chapter II

GENERAL DIRECTION FOR THE MANAGEMENT OF INFANTS

Before commencing a description of the most common diseases of infants and children, we think it necessary to offer some general instructions on the management of early infancy, touching on points which may appear to be of only minor importance, but which have a most important bearing on the *prevention* of infantile disease and mortality.

THE NEWLY-BORN INFANT

As an illustration of helpless weakness, nothing can exceed that which an infant presents at birth. The little thing requires aid of every kind, and if abandoned it soon perishes.

If an infant be born before the doctor's arrival, it should receive the attentions pointed out in the section on "Labour" in *The Lady's Manual* (Sec. 57). If the child is healthy and strong, it will cry vigorously ; for the transition from a condition of unconscious repose, in a bland fluid, at a temperature of 98° Fahr., to the contact of rough clothes, and a comparatively cold temperature, cannot be agreeable. The act of crying helps to fill the lungs with air, and thus the functions of breathing and pulmonary circulation become established.

As soon as breathing has fairly commenced, and the navel-string been tied, the infant should be enveloped in soft warmed flannel, and, everything being ready beforehand, immediately washed, and as quickly as possible. *Immediately*, for the skin requires cleansing from the tenacious fluid which adheres to it at birth, in order that healthy transpiration may be established. A newborn child is often allowed to remain a long time before it is washed, and even then it is not always washed *quickly* and skillfully, so that it shivers, and its skin becomes blue before it is placed by its mother's side.   **The First Wash**

Before commencing the process of washing, the eyelids should be carefully wiped with a piece of moist soft linen, then the rest of the body should be cleansed by means of a fine sponge, with warm water and a little soap,* and carefully dried with a soft warmed towel. If the unctuous matter be considerable or very adhesive, a little fresh lard rubbed upon the skin previously to the application of the soap and water will render its entire removal an easy operation. As soon as the cleansing is completed, a little violet powder—finely powdered, scented starch—may be dusted lightly on the surface, especially in the creases of the joints.

This is to be done by folding a piece of soft linen into four or six thicknesses, about six inches by three, and cutting a hole through the centre for the remnant of the cord, winding around it a strip of soft linen ; then one half of the folded linen should be doubled over the other half, so that the portion of cord lies between the folds, and directed upwards towards the

---

* Common scented soaps should be carefully avoided ; a glycerine soap or the common primrose coloured are the best.

chest ; the whole is to be kept in apposition by a band, about four inches wide, passed gently around the child's abdomen, and worn till the remnant of the cord comes away, which is usually within six days. All the linen thus used should be rendered surgically clean by scorching before a fire. The raw surface left after separation must be protected with scorched liner until completely healed over some seven days later. If any signs of inflammation or suppuration show themselves, bathe with weak lysol (an eggspoonful to a pint of warm water) and give *Hepar Sulph.* internally.   **Dressing the Navel***

The infant must never sleep in the mother's bed, but in a cradle or cot by her side, and every care must be taken to keep it warm.

It is affirmed by some nurses that until the third day after labour the breasts contain no milk, and that a substitute— gruel or some other farinaceous preparation—is necessary. In the great majority of cases, milk or a kind of milk sufficient for all the requirements of the infant, is present on the first day, and the only thing necessary to be done is to apply the child's mouth to the nipple. Should there be no milk at the moment, the suction of the infant, which is the natural mammary stimulant, will hasten the secretion ; while the suction promotes the necessary uterine contractions which are favourable to the mother and also lessens the chance of what is called "milk fever." The infant should be put to the breast every four hours during the first day, and somewhat oftener on subsequent days until the milk comes freely. If the child cannot get enough and is unhappy in consequence, it should have sweetened water several times a day, best given after unsuccessful attempts upon the mother. No other food should

---

* See also "Ruptured Navel," Chapter VIII.

be given. When the flow of milk has been fairly established, the child should be put to the breast every three hours, the breasts being used alternately. If during the first two or three days of life the infant's temperature rises to over 101° and there is no unhealthy appearance of the cord or other evidence of illness, the child is suffering from hunger and must be fed (see page 20).   **Milk in the Breasts the First Day**

STILL-BORN INFANTS

Children are sometimes born *apparently dead*, and if means are not quickly adopted, this condition may pass into one of real and permanent death. But so long as the heart continues to beat, even but feebly, there is a probability that well-directed efforts will be successful in exciting breathing.

Causes—Constitutional feebleness, so that the effort necessary to commence breathing cannot be made; obstructed circulation during labour by pressure or twisting of the navel-string ; too long-continued compression of the head ; tenacious muscus in the mouth and throat, preventing the entrance of air, etc.

Treatment—The navel-string should be at once divided.* Obstructive mucus should be carefully wiped away from the mouth and throat, and the general surface exposed to cold air ; an attempt should then be made to excite the function of breathing by blowing in the infant's face, sprinkling cold water with some little force on the face or chest, or alternately cold and hot, and by giving several smart blows with the hand, or

---

* It is hardly necessary to say that whenever there is serious danger, and however careful and experienced the nurse may be, the services of a medical man should be secured without loss of time.

with the corner of a towel wetted with cold water, on the buttocks, back, and chest. The back and limbs should be well rubbed, while the face is *freely exposed to the air*.

The following is another capital method of exciting breathing:—Close the infant's nostrils by the finger and thumb, press the windpipe gently backwards, and then blow into the mouth, so as to drive the air into the lungs ; afterwards press the ribs together, so that the lungs may expel the air. The process should take place about fifteen times in one minute, and if persevered in, is most likely to be successful in a short time. Meanwhile the body should lie on a flat surface, and be well rubbed with warm flannels, and the head not suffered during these efforts to fall on the chest.

If these means are not successful, the infant should be plunged into a warm bath, 98° Fahr., or what is agreeable to the back of the hand. If the sudden plunge does not excite breathing, it will be no use keeping the infant in the bath beyond a minute of two, and Dr. Marshall Hall's ready method may then be tried as follows :—

"Place the infant on its face ; turn the body gently, but completely, *on the side and a little beyond,* and then on the face, alternately ; repeating these measures deliberately, efficiently, and perseveringly, fifteen times in the minute only."

A few physical facts with regard to the normal infant should be borne in mind. The anterior fontanelle on the head should close between eighteen months and two years. A depressed state of the fontanelle is an indication of a feeble state of health. A child should begin to hold up its head at three or four months, and to walk from twelve to eighteen months. The milk teeth come through between six months and three years, and the permanent set start at six years. Babies should be weighed regularly, as this is the most important test of progress. Dr. Hutchison has pointed out the multiples of seven to be noted in regard to the normal child's weight : at birth 7 lbs, at four months 14 lbs., at twelve month 21 lbs., at six years 42 lbs., and at twelve years 84 lbs.

WASHING AND BATHING

Cleanliness is of great importance to the healthy growth of children. An infant in health should have a tepid bath twice in twenty-four hours—morning and evening. The best method is to dip the baby into a bath of tepid water, while the head is supported by the hand and arm of the nurse, and then have the whole surface of the skin rapidly rubbed with a soft soaped sponge or piece of flannel ; next again immerse the body in the bath, and then quickly and thoroughly dry with a fine warm towel. During warm weather, tepid bathing should not be continued beyond one or two months, after which it should *gradually* give place to cold. *Feeble* infants may require tepid bathing somewhat longer. For children born in the winter, the lukewarm bath may be continued till the return of warm weather, when the change to cold would be made. Except as above stated, warm bathing is to be emphatically condemned. The use of cold water, on the other hand, affords a great protection to children against excessive sensibility to atmospheric changes. But no child should have a cold bath oftener than once a day.   **Cold Water Bathing**

The care of the eyes is a subject of such enormous importance that we must notice it a little more particularly. The following is from *The Prescriber*, by Dr. John H. Clarke :—   **The eyes**

"Immediately after birth the nurse must wash the infant's eyes with the greatest possible care, removing all traces of mucus. For this purpose a fine linen rag, dipped in clean water, may be used. Beginning at the outer corner, the eyelids are gently wiped from side to side, until all traces of mucus are removed, and the eyelids remain perfectly clean. Sponges must never be used. As soon as the child's eyes are thus washed, cleaned and dried, the nurse is to wash her own hands most carefully in water with which some carbolic acid, Condy's fluid, or other disinfectant has been mixed. If in the first few days after birth signs of inflammation appear—redness, swelling, and sticking together of the lids—the greatest care must be taken. If from any reason the doctor cannot be in attendance immediately, the nurse must herself clean the eyes in the following manner :—A perfectly clean and very soft piece of linen is moistened with tepid water; any excess of water is then squeezed out. The muco-purulent discharge between the eyelids is wiped off very gently—without scrubbing or scratching; special attention being paid to the inner corner of the eyelid where the mucus particularly accumulates. After repeatedly rinsing the linen in clean water, the ball of the eye is gently raised by means of the thumb placed on the eyelid immediately above the lashes, but without making any undue pressure. The muco-purulent matter which escapes is removed with the rag as often as it appears. In the next place, the lower eyelid is drawn down with the forefinger, and also wiped with great care. If the eyelids stick together, they must be moistened with water until separation takes place without any effort. The water used in cleansing the eyes must be perfectly pure; no milk or soap is to be mixed with it. *Medical Treatment—Argent.-nit.* 3, 2h.; after well washing, a drop of a solution of *Arg.-nit* (two grains to the ounce) to be introduced into the eye."

THE WARM BATH

The temperature of the water for a *hot* bath should be about 98° to 100°, or what can be agreeably borne by the back of the hand, and for a *warm* bath, about 90°, the temperature should be *fully maintained*, by additions of hot water carefully poured down the side of the bath till the child is taken out. The bath should be given in front of a good fire, and a warm blanket be in readiness to wrap the child in directly when it leaves the bath.

The warm bath, given for five or ten minutes, is of great value in many affections of children, especially in febrile diseases; in spasmodic affections of the bowels, or bladder; in Prurigo, Tetanus, and in Convulsions. In the last-mentioned disease, a towel or sponge squeezed out of cold water should also be applied to the head for two or three minutes.

CLOTHING

Besides adapting it to the season, the clothing should be loose, soft, light, warm, arranged to fit without pins, and to cover the legs, arms, and neck. After the separation of the navel-string, a belt, stays, etc., are unnecessary.

When a baby is divested of its long clothes, it is in danger of being insufficiently clad, the danger increasing when it can run alone and is more exposed to atmospheric influences. It cannot be too strongly impressed upon those who have the charge of children, that the practice of leaving parts of the body exposed which, in the case of adults, it is found necessary to clothe warmly, especially the lower limbs and abdomen, is a frequent cause of Colic, Diarrhoea, and perhaps more serious diseases.

Warmth is of prime importance for children of all ages, and especially so for newly-born infants. Warm clothing should cover the whole body. But in hot weather it is necessary to keep children cool, for Diarrhoea and other summer complaints may be thus to a great extent avoided. Excess of clothing, night or day, is to be guarded against, and the use of flannel or wool in contact with the skin is unnecessary except in rheumatic children. The clothing, too, should be scrupulously *clean*, and all soiled and wet articles immediately changed. Caps are unnecessary; the aim should be rather to "keep the head cool and the feet warm." In all cases the night clothing should be looser and less warm than that worn in the day. It is also important that the dress should not impede the free movement of the limbs, or exert pressure on the digestive, breathing, or circulatory organs.

SLEEP

It is advisable that children should sleep apart from the mother or nurse, in a cot, care being taken that they are warmly but not excessively covered. Not only in fants, but children of both sexes should, if possible, sleep

Child Should Sleep Alone

During the first few months after its birth a healthy infant spends the chief part of its time in sleep. Even up to about the third year a midday sleep is beneficial.   **Amount of Sleep**

He should be fed, and put to bed, at stated hours, as regularity is of the greatest importance in all matters pertaining to children.

Regularity

When the time for sleep arrives, infants should be placed directly into their cot awake; the unnecessary and objectionable habit of rocking or nursing them to sleep in the arms should never be formed. Neither should ordinary footsteps, speaking, or other moderate sounds be avoided, but the infant should be accustomed to sleep under such conditions.   **No Rocking**

All the so-called soothing remedies, syrups, cordials, spirits, or sleeping drops, should be strictly avoided, containing as they do, to a greater or less extent, *Opium* in some of its forms. These sleeping mixtures inflict an incalculable amount of mischief on health, and largely swell infantile mortality. No medicines to promote sleep should ever be given except such as are prescribed in the section (page 98) on "Sleeplessness." Dummy teats should not be allowed. They cannot be kept clean, and they are apt to spoil the shape of the jaws and possibly help to cause adenoids.   **Sleeping Medicines**

Pure fresh air is of extreme importance to children during sleep. Nurseries should be as spacious and airy as possible. The practice of shutting bedroom doors is objectionable, if the children can be protected from draught. A great advantage to health is secured by separate night and day nurseries; but when this is impracticable, the children should be out of the nursery a great deal, and every opportunity seized for promoting ventilation, by opening doors and windows at all suitable times. Ideal ventilation, at any rate in cold weather, is secured by the combination of a fire and open windows.   **Ventilation**

OPEN-AIR EXERCISE

Children require fresh air and sunlight as much as plants and flowers do; and as the later are colourless and imperfect if excluded from direct sunshine, so children who live in places where light does not abundantly enter are pale and feeble. In fine weather, an infant over a month old should be taken out at least twice a day; the only precaution necessary being that it should be sufficiently clothed. In warm, sunny weather, the more it is in the open air the better, if care be observed to protect the head from the hot sun. In shout, a child should almost live out of doors during suitable weather. Plenty of exercise in the open air is necessary for the healthy development of the limbs and body generally. Suitable athletic games and exercises should form a part of the early education of all children, and these games and exercises should take place in the open air, except during inclement weather, when they may be carried out in spacious, well-ventilated rooms.

Chapter III

EXAMPLES OF DIETARY FOR HEALTHY CHILDREN, AT DIFFERENT AGES

In consequence of the vital importance of the diet of children, for health, for growth and development, we deem it necessary to give detailed examples of dietary adapted to infants and other children at ages when they are most likely to be improperly fed, and when the consequences of such feeding are sure to tell disastrously: namely, 1st, from birth to six months old; 2nd, from six to twelve months; 3rd, from twelve to eighteen months; and 4th, from eighteen months to two years, and upwards. As it is impossible to make one invariable rule applicable to the different constitutions and requirements of children, it is scarcely necessary to add that the quantities stated in the following arrangements are only approximative. But the amounts of farinaceous food stated will generally be found sufficient.

As the diet suitable for children *suffering from disease* is pointed out in the various following Sections of this Manual it is not described in the present Section.

FOR THE FIRST SIX MONTHS

Diet 1—We commence by stating emphatically that children who enjoy their inalienable right to maternal breast-milk, assuming this to be suitable in quality and sufficient in quantity, require *no other food*. The infant should be applied to the breast every two hours and a half during the day for about the first six weeks; afterwards only once in every three or four hours. But he should not be awakened from sleep at night to be fed. After about the first month or even earlier it will not be necessary to give the breast at all between the hours of 11 p.m. and 5 or 6 a.m. The early commencement of this arrangement is very important, as it affords the opportunity for the regular, undisturbed repose, which contributes much to the well-being of both mother and child. It is important, too, that the infant should suck from each breast alternately. Regular habits of feeding may be soon acquired; it is a great mistake and the cause of wind, Colic, and other disorders, to give the infant the breast whenever it cries, or to let it be always sucking.

It should not be too readily assumed that the mother is unable to nurse her infant. Perseverance, more meat and milk and perhaps lactagol for the mother, often work wonders. On the other hand, though there may be plenty of milk, the child may suffer from dyspepsia which is sometimes corrected by restricting the mother's food or making her take more exercise.

A nursing mother or wet-nurse does not require an extra or a rich dietary, but discrimination in selection of her food. The meal-hours should be regular, and late meals avoided. The thirst to which nursing mothers are liable is best appeased by milk-and-water, barely-water, toast-and-water, and similar beverages. Stimulants are best avoided.   **Diet for a Nursing Mother**

Diet 2—For children brought up by hand. The best substitute for mother's milk is good milk from a good dairy, diluted with boiled (not boiling) water half and half, and enriched by the addition of sugar (sugar of milk if possible) and cream. The milk should be scalded—either by heating over the flame until the first small bubbles begin to form (at 160°) or by standing for ten minutes in a vessel of boiling water (water *kept* boiling). Three-quarters of an ounce of sugar (a tablespoonful and a half) dissolved in 18 ounces of boiled water may be mixed as wanted with an equal quantity of the scalded milk and then given from a modern feeding-bottle with a simple rubber teat. Avoid all tubes. Be sure that the hole in the teat is the right size so that the child gets the milk neither too fast nor too slowly. The bottle and teat should be thoroughly washed out after each meal and kept in a basin of cold water. The child's mouth ought also to be cleansed out with fresh water after every feed. Under three months the child should receive 2½ oz. of the milk mixture every two and half hours, at three months 3 oz. every three hours. The interval then remains the same up to six months, but the amount is increased an ounce every month. At six months the interval should be four hours, and by that time the half-and-half proportion should give way to two of milk and one of water.

Diet 3— Children that cannot be breast-fed are often very difficult to feed by the bottle. If the half-and-half milk mixture just described is not digested, try first *citrating* the milk by the addition of a grain of sodium citrate to every ounce of milk and then diluting with water as before, if the child still cannot digest the milk, try *condensed milk* (Nestlés), adding a teaspoonful of it to three table-spoonfuls of water, and further adding (because of the deficiency of fat) a teaspoonful of cream to each feed. It may even be necessary to *peptonize* the milk. Fairchild's peptonizing powders are the best known, and directions for their use are supplied with them. In some cases milk in any form disagrees and then *whey* must be tried, fortified by Mellin's food, (follow the Mellin directions, substituting whey for the milk-and-water).

In all cases of artificial feeding, and in many of breast feeding, it is in the highest degree desirable to give the child fruit-juice (juice of oranges, grapes, etc.), diluted with water and sweetened, a teaspoonful two or three times a day. This helps the bowels and also supplies some of the *vitamins* or accessory food factors that the system requires.

DIET FROM NINE TO TWELVE MONTHS CHILD

Diet 4—Weaning should take place normally at the end of the ninth month. If the mother's health flags in any way or if her milk ceases to satisfy the infant's requirements, weaning may have to take place earlier. It should not under any circumstances be delayed much beyond the tenth month. "Never wean a child in hot weather if you can avoid it" (R. Hutchison), for fear of epidemic Diarrhoea. By this time it will be possible to introduce starch into the child's dietary. Indeed, the appearance of the milk teeth is probably a sign that starch can now be digested. From the time the child has two or three teeth he should be encouraged to gnaw a hard crust or bite at a whole (raw) apple. This promotes the development of the jaws and lessens the likelihood of adenoids developing.

Diet 5—For a weaned child above nine months old the following arrangement may be adopted.

First Meal, 7 a.m.—A breakfast-cupful of prepared food, such a Chapman's, Mellin's or Allenbury's No. 3, prepared as directed on the tin, or Robinson's groats with milk. If the bowels are confined at any time, a rather larger proportion of the food, and less of the milk, should be used; or the reverse if the bowels are relaxed.

Second Meal, 10.30 a.m.—A breakfast-cupful of milk. A teaspoonful of lime-water may be added when the milk has appeared to produce discomfort.

Third Meal, 2 p.m. — The yoke of one egg, well beaten up in a teacupful of milk. Beef tea* occasionally as a change.

Fourth Meal, 5.30 p.m. — Same as the first.

Fifth Meal, 10 p.m. — Same as the second. Water to be given freely between meals.

No food of any kind should be given between the meals, which should, therefore, be made sufficiently large to meet the requirements of the system, always stopping short of over-repletion. A healthy child from ten to twelve months old requires from a pint and a half to a quart of milk in the twenty-four hours.

FROM TWELVE TO EIGHTEEN MONTHS OLD

Diet 6—*First Meal, 7.30 a.m.* — A rusk or a slice of stale Hovis bread with a breakfast-cupful of new milk. The bread may be soaked in the milk; but if the child has teeth, it should

---

* BEEF-TEA may be made in the following way : Put half a pound (or a pound, according to the strength required) of rump steak cut up into small pieces, into a covered enamelled saucepan with one pint of cold water. Let this stand in a cold or cool place for four or five hours, and then by the side of a fire till the temperature should approach but not reach the boiling-point. It is then fit for use.

The meat used should be *freshly-slain,* and divested beforehand of all fat or gristle; otherwise a greasy taste is given to the beef-tea, which cannot be afterwards removed by skimming. Only *enamelled* saucepans should be used. In re-warming beef-tea which has been left to cool, care must be taken to warm it only up to the point at which it is be served. On no account should it be allowed to boil.

When children, from long use of it, become tried of beef-tea, it may be seasoned with some vegetable product—celery, or celery-seeds, which should be strained off before using—when, possessing an entirely new flavour, it will generally be eaten with zest.

be well masticated dry, and milk taken in sipc. The teeth and gums are improved by proper employment. See the Section 62, "Decay of the Teeth."

Second Meal, 11 a.m.—A drink of milk, with a plain biscuit or thin slice of Hovis bread-and-butter, or bread-and-dripping.

Third Meal, 1.30 p.m.—A pudding like the one recommended for the third meal in Diet 6. Or, as a variety, a teacupful of good beef-tea (a pound of meat to the pint) or of beef-gravy or mutton- or chicken-both or marmite, with rusk or stale bread. A good table-spoonful of light farinaceous pudding with baked apple or stewed prunes may follow the beef-tea.

Fourth Meal, 6 p.m.—Same as the first.

In cases of debility, or when there exists any exhausting discharge, a little milk may be given at about 10 p.m. But in good health nothing is required after 6 p.m. The sooner a child becomes accustomed to sleep all night without food the better. When however, he wakes in the morning, refreshed by his night's rest, he should not be compelled to remain fasting for an hour or more, but his breakfast should be preparely early.

FROM EIGHTEEN MONTHS TO THREE YEARS OLD AND UPWARDS

Diet 7—*First Meal, 7.30 a.m.*— A breakfast-cupful of fine oatmeal porridge and milk. Lightly boiled egg. A rusk or a good slice of stale whole-meal bread.

Second Meal, 11 a.m.—A cup of milk.

Third Meal, 1.30 p.m.—A small slice of underdone roast mutton, or fish, or chicken, one well-mashed potato, with a little gravy as it runs from the cut surfaces of the joint. For drink, water or milk-and-water.

Fourth Meal, 6 p.m.—A breakfast-cupful of milk and whole meal bread-and-butter; occasionally some plain cake. A healthy child, after the age of eighteen months, should sleep from 6 p.m. to 6 a.m. without waking and require nothing beyond the above.

Special care must be taken to see that the child chews properly.

The morning and evening meals should always consist principally of milk. Tea and coffee should be entirely withheld from young children. Indeed, these beverages are better not given at all till after adult age. Cocoa, however, properly prepared, is a suitable beverage at any period of life after infancy, and may often, made with milk and water, replace pure milk where this seems to cause sickness, pale stools, loss of appetite, and even slight fever. Sweets should be allowed in the strictest moderation—good toffee or chocolate once a week, the child being required to brush the teeth immediately after.

Vitamins, of which one hears so much nowadays, are food elements or "accessory food factors" which are essential to health and nutrition. The three chief vitamins are numbered A, B and C. Vitamin A is abundant in animal fats, and therefore the child who has abundant butter, dripping, milk, and egg-yolk is well supplied. Vitamin B is abundant in whole meal cereals—hence the desirability of an early introduction of whole meal bread into the diet; also in egg-yolk and marmite. Vitamin C is contained in milk and potato. It is also, and most abundantly, contained in fresh fruit and in greens cooked for a short time. From two years these articles should be added to the diet, especially oranges, apples, grape-fruit, tomato (these are cooked, not by boiling, but *always by steaming*, which preserves the precious salts of the vegetables).

Part II

DISEASES OF INFANTS AND CHILDREN, AND THEIR HOMOEOPATHIC AND GENERAL TREATMENT

Chapter I

ACUTE SPECIFIC DISEASES

SCARLET FEVER (Febris Rubra)—SCARLATINA

The *Mortality* of Scarlet fever is very large, and the disease destroying every year in this country the lives of some twenty thousand persons. During the same time it more or less completely disables, often for a long period, a hundred thousand others. Yet, judging by the results that have been effected by disinfection, separation, and preventive treatment, by far the larger amount of this waste of life and costly sickness might be averted.

Scarlet fever is chiefly prevalent in children, especially from the second to the fifth year of life. It is by no means infrequent during the second year, and even occurs before the end of the first, although infants a few months old seem to enjoy a special immunity. We have often attended families in which all the children have been suffering from the disease except the baby, who, crowing and

smiling all the time, was the only one unaffected. After the
tenth year the susceptibility rapidly diminishes. The
common notion that *Scarlatina* is a mild, and *Scarlet fever* a
severe form of the disease, is incorrect, for the terms are
synonymous.

Varieties—There are three varieties, or, more correctly,
degrees of intensity; for though it is convenient to speak of
Scarlatina simplex, S. anginosa, and *S. maligna,* they are but
one disease, manifesting different degrees of severity.
Exposure to the infection of *S. simplex* may give rise to an
attack of *S. maligna* and the reverse. The same organs are
affected, the same functions are disturbed, and the same
secondary diseases follows in each case. The characteristics
of each variety are as follows:—1. *S. simplex*— A scarlet rash
with moderate fever and slightly enlarged and inflamed
tonsils. 2. *S. anginosa,* those of *S. simplex* in an aggravated
form, with a more severe affection of the throat, and
swelling of the submaxillary glands. 3. *S. maligna.* The rash
is of a dark-red, colour, often haemorrhagic, and comes out
later than in the other varieties, and often imperfectly or
irregularly; there is no ulceration of the throat or glandular
enlargement, but profound taxaemia, shown by a very high
temperature, very rapid and feeble by a very high
temperature, very rapid and feeble pulse, restlessness and
delirium soon giving place to coma. Death may occur
within thirty-six hours.

Mode of Propagation—Although we are ignorant of the
origin of Scarlet fever, we know that it spreads by infection,
and that most rapidly and persistently. It is by no means
necessary to have direct contact with a patient, or to imbibe
or touch anything that has been directly contaminated by
him—it is not even necessary to be in the same room, in
order to take the disease. The poison rapidly diffuses itself
throughout the whole house unless stringent preventive

disinfecting measures are adopted, and no inmate can be said to be safe unless he has previously had the disease, and even then he is not absolutely so. The poison may be conveyed in milk. The unseen germs, which no microscope can detect, are not only very rapid and fatal in their action, they are also very tenacious. They lurk in all kinds of places, and cling to everything. The clothes of attendants as well as of the patient, the bedding, furniture, and walls of the rooms, persistently retain the poison. And they have been known to communicate the disease after an interval of one or two years.

General Symptoms—Scarlatina has an incubation period of two to five days. It commences with the ordinary symptoms of fever—chills, shivering, hot skin, frontal headache, rapid pulse, nausea, vomiting, thirst, and *sore throat*. The last-named symptom is generally the first complained of by the patient.

After a short time the pulse becomes very quick, often in children 120 to 140 in the minute. In about forty-eight hours after the occurrence of these symptoms, the rash comes out, first on the breast, then on the neck, face, body, and over the great joints and limbs, till the whole body is covered with it.

The eruption usually fades away in the same order. Its appearance is a *bright-scarlet efflorescence*, consisting of innumerable smooth spots, not raised above the skin, having the colour and semblance of a boiled lobster-shell. The colour disappears on pressure, but immediately returns on its removal.

The tongue at first is coated with a creamy fur, the tip and edges are red, the papillae are red and raised, giving it a peculiar strawberry-like appearance. This is always exhibited in the course of the disorder, and not infrequently at its commencement. The tongue afterwards becomes preternaturally clean and raw-looking. A diffused redness, sometimes of a dark claret colour, covers the mouth, fauces, etc., which disappears as the febrile symptoms and rash subside. On about the fifth day the efflorescence generally begins to decline, and by about the eighth or ninth entirely disappears, leaving the patient prostrate.

During a period of uncertain length, the outer skin comes off as scurf, or moulded masses are thrown off especially from the hands and feet. The diseases does not, however, always pursue this uniform course. In the exceedingly dangerous form we have described, the eruption is either entirely wanting, or lived and partial. In the anginose variety the mucous membranes are threatened with gangrene, the glands and even the cellular tissue of the neck are very much swollen, membranous exudation as in Diphtheria may form in the pharynx and spread upto into the nose, constitutional disturbance is profound and the child may quickly die. Short of this there may be extensive suppuration and sloughing in the tissues of the neck.

Treatment—At the commencement of the illness, or before its true nature is recognized, the febrile symptoms may be modified by a dose of *Acon.* every two or three hours. When the characteristic redness of the skin or throat shows itself, *Bell.* should be administered in a similar manner; or if the fever continue high, the two medicines may be given alternately, at intervals of two hours. If the case be one of *S. simplex* no other medicine will probably be needed, until it is on the decline, when *Sulph.* should be taken night and morning for two or three days. In *S. anginosa, Acon.* will hardly be needed, *Apis* or *Mercurius* will have to take a place of Bell., and, if the heat of skin or restlessness be considerable, in alternation with *Gelseminum.* In *S. maligna, Ailan.* or *Ammon.-Carb.* will be more especially called for.

Dangers—Pneumonia, Bronchitis, Diphtheria, and inflammation of the larynx may arise during the course of the disease. Phthisis, Diphtheria, disease of the glands and bones, Chronic Ophthalmia, Otorrhoea, and skin diseases may follow the attack.

Treatment—In the early state *Acon.* should be given every two or three hours to subdue the fever. As soon as the symptoms peculiar to the disease manifest themselves, *Puls.* must be administrated alone every two or three hours, or, if necessary, in alternation with the *Acon.* at intervals of two hours. The cough almost invariably attendant upon the disease may be mitigated by a dose or two of *Bell.* or *Hyos.* If the eye-symptoms are very troublesome, great smarting and intolerance of light, they should be bathed every few hours with a lotion of *Euphrasia*, in the proportion of a teaspoonful to a teacupful of water.

Indications for the Above and other Remedies

Remedies—*Aconitum*—Febrile symptoms at the outset or during the process of the disease. A dose every third or fourth hour.

Ant.-Tart.—Where there are decided bronchial symptoms, or nausea with white-furred tongue.

Belladonna—Sore throat, *dry, barking cough*, etc.; headache, drowsiness, or restlessness, and tendency to *delirium*.

Bryonia—Imperfect or suppressed eruption, stitching pains in the chest, difficult breathing, *cough*, etc. For a *sudden recession* of the eruption, this remedy, or *Acon.*, may be given every half hour.

Euphrasia—May be called for when the discharge of tears is profuse.

Gelseminum—Slow development or retrocession of the rash.

Mercurius Sol. 3x and *Cor.* 3x—Ulcerous, glandular, or dysenteric affections.

Phosphorus—Dry, hollow cough, with tendency to Pneumonia.

Pulsatilla—Almost *specific*, especially for the symptoms of cold, gastric derangement, phlegm in the chest, etc. It is most useful after the fever has been modified by *Aconite*, and rarely any other remedies are required.

Sulphur—After the eruption has completed its natural course, and the other remedies are discontinued. It may avert secondary diseases. A dose morning and night, for several days.

Secondary Disease—Measles is often succeeded by diseases of the lungs, eyes, ears, bones, or some affection of the skin. These are often far more serious than the malady itself, and generally require professional treatment. They may often be prevented by the administration of *Sulphur*, or other remedy indicated. Sequelae are infrequent after homoeopathic treatment. If, however, after the decline of the eruption, the patient retains a temperature above 100°F., some complicating disturbance may be suspected.

Remedies for the Sequelae

Inflammatory Affections of the Eyelids—Acon., Bell., Merc.-Cor., Sulph.

Purulent Discharge from Ear, or Deafness—Hep.-Sulph., Merc., Plus., Sil., Sulph.

Glandular Swelling—Calc.-Carb., Iod., Lyc., Merc.

Chest Complication—Ars., Hep.-Sulph., Kali Bich., Spong.

Cutaneous Eruptions—Iod., Ars., Sulph.

Styes—Bell., Calc.-Carb., Puls., Sulph.

Consumption—*Wasting, Cough, Hoarseness, etc.*—Ars., Dros., Hep.-S., Phos., Spong., and Cod-liver oil.

Measles and Consumptions—Tubercular disease of the lungs, or more often of the bowels, or of the bronchial glands, or miliary tuberculosis (in which very minute tubercles are seeded over, it may be, several organs), are by no means infrequent sequels in delicate children. When, therefore, a child makes but slow or imperfect recovery from Measles and the temperature remains up, a grave constitutional disease may be suspected, and no time should be lost in obtaining professional advice.

Accessories—When Measles occur before weaning, the infant may refuse to suck, in consequence of the closure of the nasal passages ; resort must then be had to artificial feeding with the spoon. *Cold* water, gum-water, barely-water, etc., are the best drinks. No stimulants. As the fever abates, milk diet may be given, gradually returning to more nourishing food. Should the eruption be imperfectly developed, or recede suddenly, the child should be put into a hot bath (see page 15), or be packed in a blanket wrung out or hot water. During the whole of the illness the wet-pack and tepid sponging, with careful drying, should be employed once or twice a day, and the linen should be frequently changed. We have emphasized "frequent change of linen," as there exists a widespread prejudice among mothers and nurses against clean clothes in this disease. The patient should be kept warm in bed, with the room equably warmed to about 65°, but light and well ventilated, a shawl or curtain being so suspended as to protect the eyes. A fire, except in the very height of summer. After the disease has subsided the patient should be warmly clad (in flannel), and taken into the open air *frequently* when the weather is fine. But he must not go out of doors too soon, or be at all exposed to cold, draughts, or wet.

Preventive—*Puls.* every morning and *Acon.* every evening for a week or ten days, during the prevalence of Measles.

Indications for the above and other Remedies

Aconitum—Hot skin, thirst, headache, restlessness, and other febrile symptoms.

Ailanthus Gland—*Maliganant* Scarlatina, with purple or nearly suppressed rash, foetid discharge from the nostrils, cracking at the angles of the mouth, etc. It should be given directly when unfavourable symptoms are observed, and frequently repeated until improvement ensues. This is indicated by increase of the eruption, by its assuming a scarlet colour, and by diminished circulatory and nervous disturbances.

Ammon.-Carb—Very decided physical and mental prostration.

Apis.—Urgent throat symptoms, and when there is more oedema than ulceration.

Arsenicum—*Severe prostration, excessive thirst,* cold clammy sweats, frequent weak pulse, threatened diarrhoea.

Belladonna—Is specific in, and exerts a direct power over, Scarlet fever in its simple form. When the eruption is of a *scarlet* colour the disease will frequently yield to the action of this remedy without the aid of any other.

Gelseminum—Imperfect eruption, nervous restlessness, *remittent* symptoms.

Mercurius Sol. 6—Inflamed, swollen, or ulcerated throat; difficult swallowing; *copious saliva,* ulcers in the mouth; acrid discharge from the nostrils.

Muriatic Acid—*Malignant sore throat,* with extreme depression, tremors, etc.

Sulphur—When the disease is on the decline, to prevent secondary complaints: a dose morning and night for several days.

Veratrum Viride—Severe *cerebral disturbance,* vomiting, and very rapid pulse.

Additional Remedies—*Ant.-Tart.* (in the first state, if attended with convulsions, cold sweat, difficult breathing or vomiting); *Coffea or Hyos.* (restlessness and sleeplessness) *Cupr.-Acet.* (sudden retrocession of the rash); *Digit.* (little urine, dropsy); *Arum triph.* (ulceration of throat, raw condition of nostrils, lips, and mouth); *Crotalus or Ecchinacea* (*S. anginosa* or *S. maligna*); *Hepar Sulph.* (to prevent after-effects of Scarlet fever).

Secondary Diseases (*Sequelae*)—The following are the chief:—1. Inflammatory swelling of the glands of the neck, which in scrofulous children may attain a large size, suppurate, and the pus burrow under the muscles of the neck. *Merc., Hepar S.,* and *Calc.,* are the chief remedies. 2. The inflammation of the throat may be extended along the *Eustachian tubes*, producing deafness by their obstruction, or by suppuration of the tympanum, or some other mischief of the car. The remedies recommended are *Bell., Merc., Aurum,* or *Puls.* 3. But the most frequent and dangerous sequel is Anasarca, the treatment of which will be found in Section Post-Scarlatinal Dropsy page 37.

Complete suppression of urine without dropsy is far from uncommon. It may last for several days, and terminate either in the gradual resumption of the functions of the kidneys, or in blood-poisoning, sudden Convulsions, and death.

Accessories—The patient should be placed in a separate room which can be so ventilated as to secure a copious and continual supply of *fresh air*; for the one means above all others which mitigates the virulence and infectiveness of Scarlet fever is ventilation. The room should be as free from furniture as possible. Curtains, carpets, and woolen stuffs should be removed. A fire is necessary in cold weather. Condy's fluid or carbolic acid should be freely used about the room; and a sheet across the open door, kept moist with the disinfectant, will purify the air for the patient, and lessen the infection through the house. Sponding the surface of the body with tepid water, piece by piece, moderates the great heat and allays restlessness, quiets delirium, lowers the pulse, and favours sleep. A wet bandage to the throat, when it is affected, is a sovereign remedy, and seldom fails to relieve. It should be fastened both at the back of the neck and at the top of the head, so as to protect the glands near the angles of the jaws. Inhalation of steam from hot water is useful when the throat is sore and painful. The *wet-pack*, especially at the commencement, is often most valuable, and it may be repeated several times, at a few hours' interval, as long as severe febrile symptoms continue; but it requires to be administered by an experienced person. When the eruption is slow in coming out, or is suddenly suppressed, the child should have a hot bath (see Section 7) or be packed in a blanket wrung out of hot water. During convalescence, warm clothing, including flannel is necessary; and subsequently a change of air, if possible to the seaside. The patient must not, however, go out too early, as secondary symptoms are of frequent occurrence from neglect of this precaution.

In all cases of *S. Anginosa,* or indeed in all but the mildest cases of Scarlatina, a toilet of the throat should be instituted. The simplest is swabbing the throat with carbolic oil (1 in 10). The best method is that of Caiger (*practitioner's Encyclopedia of Medicine and Surgery,* p. 72). "A four-ounce rubber ball syringe, the nozzle of which should be short to avoid risk of damaging the palate . . . is introduced between the biscuspid or molar teeth, passed over the surface of the tongue, and then directed backwards, so that the stream of fluid impinges on the tonsils and back of the pharynx, the patient's head being meanwhile bent over a basin to catch the escaping lotion . . . three drachms of strong hydrochloric acid are poured upon six drachms of powdered chlorate of potash and quart of water gradually added, the vessel being frequently . . . shaken up . . . This solution should be diluted with an equal volume of either hot or iced water, and about a pint of fluid used on each occasion."

Diet—During the whole course of the fever, milk, either alone or with plain or soda-water, thin gruel, sago, arrowroot, yolk of egg beaten up with cold milk, grapes, oranges, and cooked fruits, should be the staple diet. The drink may consist of cold water gum-water, weak lemonade, etc., in small quantities as frequently as desired. As soon as the fever subsides, the patient may gradually and cautiously return to more substantial food. Stimulants are rarely necessary except in malignant cases, when wine, brandy, Liebig's extract of beef, beef-tea, etc., may be given *regularly* in frequent small doses, under medical care.

Preventive Measures—1. *To be adopted by the unaffected*: During the prevalence of Scarlatina, a dose of *Belladonna* should be given, morning and night, to children who have not had the disease. The first or second dilution of the tincture is best for this purpose. Should the disease occur notwithstanding this treatment, its severity will be much mitigated. The author has great faith in the virtue of *Belladonna* thus used, both as the result of his own experiences, and from the testimonies of numerous *confrères* and correspondents. 2. *To be adopted by the attendants upon the invalid*: The attendant should have as little intercourse with the other members of the household as possible. She should wear over her ordinary clothes an overall which she can readily take off and hang on a peg before she leaves the sick-chamber. She should also dip her hands into a disinfectant after touching the patient, and especially before quitting the room. Condy's fluid or Chloride of Lime—one tablespoonful of either to about a gallon of water—is usually employed for this purpose. All excretions from the invalid should be disinfected with the Chloride of Lime solution, and disposed of at once. All washing appreal that has been used

F-4

by the patient should, on its removal, be immediately placed in a vessel containing a sufficient quantity of either of the above disinfectants, and be put out of doors as soon as possible, and afterwards boiled in the disinfectant. Woolen clothes, bedding, etc., that do not admit of being boiled, should either be burnt or fumigated by burning a sulphur candle, procurable at any oilman's. The sick-chamber itself, when the patient is permitted to leave it, should be disinfected in a similar way, doors, windows and fireplaces having been securely closed.

POST-SCARLATINAL DROPSY
(Acute Tubular Nephritis)

Homoeopathists may rejoice in the fact that under homoeopathic treatment this grave sequel of Scarlet fever is neither so frequent nor so intractable as in allopathic practice.

Symptoms—About the twelfth day after the subsidence of the fever, the subcutaneous areolar tissue becomes infiltrated with serous fluid; there is often frequent desire to pass water, which is scanty and high-coloured or smoky-looking or bloody, and albuminous. If examined by a microscope, the urine is seen to contain renal tube-casts. The pulse is quick, the temperature raised, it may be to 103°, the skin dry; the child is thirsty; and the body, face, and limbs are pale and oedematous. Occasionally the cavities of the body are more or less filled with fluid. When the cavity of the chest is invaded, there are the following symptoms—short, difficult breathing, violent action of the heart, increasing distress and lividity of the face, often followed by death. Occasionally the kidney complication exists from the outset of Scarlet fever, and is rather a form of the disease than a sequel.

Treatment—*Ars., Canth.,* and *Terebinth,* are the most useful medicines. *Canth.* and *Terebinth.* have actually produced acute nephritis. A dose of the one selected should be given every three hours.

Indications for the above and other Remedies

Apis.—*Rapid general aedema;* pale colour of the skin; scanty, high-coloured urine; swelling of the tonsils, difficulty of swelling.

Arsenicum—Scanty, dark-coloured or bloody urine, with general aedema and *prostration*.

Bryonia—Is said to be useful in the same cases. It is probably indicated when the Dropsy has followed exposure to cold, and there are muscular pains present.

Cantharis—For symptoms similar to those under *Arsenicum*, and with pain in passing water.

Terebinth—Scanty, *reddish*, or dark urine.

Additional Remedies—*Apocyn.-Can., Digitalis, Ferrum, Helleborus,* and *Hepar Sulph.*

Accessories—Warm baths, or sponging the body with warm water, the wet-pack, and drinking cold water are of the first importance; they facilitate excretion by the skin, and relieve the congested kidneys. The free action of the skin in the treatment of Scarlet fever is the most effectual means for preventing Post-scarlatinal Dropsy. Nothing secures this so thoroughly as the *wet-pack*. A nourishing, digestible diet is also essential to meet the exhaustion which usually exists. Finally, change of air is of great value.

MEASLES
(Morbilli)

Measles is a disease of childhood, in itself not serious, but liable, from want of care and especially exposure to chill, to be complicated or followed by Broncho-Pneumonia, an extremely serious condition which may itself go on to Tuberculosis.

Mode of Propagation—Infection. No susceptible person can remain in the same room or house with an infected person without risk of taking the disease; and it is almost impossible to isolate it in large establishments or schools. It is propagated, even after a considerable time has elapsed, by infected clothing, bedding, furniture or wall-paper. Infection only ceases when the peeling off of the skin is quite complete, and when all the clothing and surroundings of the patient have been thoroughly disinfected. It is strongest during the eruptive state, and especially at the early part of this state.

Symptoms—After about ten or fourteen days, the period of incubation, the disease is ushered in with the symptoms of a *Catarrh*—sneezing, running from the nose, red, swollen, and watery eyes, a hoarse harsh *cough*, languor, and *fever*, which increase in intensity. About the fourth day of the illness the *eruption* begins, and appears in three successive crops, on the face and neck, on the body, and lastly on the legs. It is in the form of small circular spots, resembling flea-bites, which multiply and coalesce into blotches of a more or less crescentic form, slightly raised above the surrounding skin, so as to be felt, particularly on the face, which is often a good deal swollen. It is like raspberry in colour, and turns white for an instant under pressure; a dark purple is a bad sign. It is two or three days in coming out, and remains at least three days. The fever then abates, and a bran-like scurf is gradually thrown off the skin. As the rash declines, diarrhoea sometimes occurs: this, unless very troublesome, should not be interfered with, as it is often beneficial.

The temperature reaches 103° or 104° on the fifth day, after which it rapidly declines.

Diagnosis—Measles can be diagnosed Measles can be diagnosed several days before the rash appears. Koplik's spots—tiny white specks surrounded by a red zone visible with a good light on the mucous membrane of the mouth in the neighbourhood of the first molar teeth—can be detected on the first and second days of illness.

Formerly this disease was confounded with Scarlet fever, but there are well-marked differences between the two, as shown below.

Tabular Differences Between Measles and Scarlet Fever

MEASLES	SCARLET FEVER
1. Rash comes out on the *fourth day*.	1. Rash appears on the *second day*.
2. *Catarrhal* symptoms are prominent— watery discharge from the eyes and nose, sneezing, harsh cough, etc.	2. Catarrhal symptoms are usually absent, but there is great *heat of the skin*, *sore throat*, and sometimes *delirium*.
3. The rash begins near the *roots of the hair*.	3. The rash begins on the *neck and face*.
4. The rash is of a *pinkish-red* of *raspberry colour*. The white streak produced by the back of the nail is not uniform, and lasts a shorter time than in Scarlet fever.	4. The eruption is of a *bright scarlet colour*, and by drawing the back of the nail over the skin a white streak is produced, which lasts two or three minutes.
5. The eruption is somewhat *rough*, so as to be felt by passing the hand over the skin, and is in crescentic groups, with natural skin between.	5. The rash usually presents no *inequalities* to sight or touch, and is so minute and closely crowded as to give the skin a *uniformly* red appearance.
6. Liquid, tender, *watery* eye.	6. A peculiar *brilliant stare*, as if the eyes were glazed.
7. The cuticle is thrown off minute portions, like fine *scales of bran*.	7. Desquamation of the cuticle is usually in *large patches*, especially from the hands and feet.
8. The most common sequeloe are diseases of the *lungs, eyes, ears*, and *skin*.	8. The most frequent *sequeloe* are *dropsy*, especially after mild cases, and *glandular swellings*.

GERMAN MEASLES (called also FALSE MEASLES, RUBELLA—German: Rötheln)

This is an infectious eruptive fever, the rash appearing during the first day of the illness, beginning on the face in rose-red spots, extending the next day to the body and limbs, subsiding with the fever on the third day, and not preceded (as Measles is) by symptoms of cold in the head, or followed (as both Measles and Scarlatina are) by shedding of the superficial skin. The disease spreads by contagion. It only attacks the same person once; but is does not protect those whom it attacks from either Scarlatina or Measles. It has a long period of incubation, usually for fortnight, but varying from seven to twenty-one days, usually its rash is the first thing noticed. There is headache, sore throat, swelling of the glands in the neck, and sharp fever. There are also, as a rule, slight catarrhal symptoms.

Diagnosis—The sudden onset of the disease distinguishes it from *Measles*, and the enlargement of the glands at the side of the neck. The appearance of the rash in distinct spots and on the face first, distinguishes it from *Scarlatina*, also the less severe sore throat, and the enlargement of the glands at the sides of the neck (and not at the angle of the jaw as in Scarlatina).

Treatment—Aconite and Belladonna should be given every hour in alternation. The general treatment is the same as for Measles; and the complications (which are very rare, the disease being attended with little danger) are to be treated, as they arise, in the same way as those of Measles and Scarlatina.

SMALLPOX (Variola)

Varieties—This, the most marked of the eruptive fevers, and one of the most malignant, loathsome, and contagious diseases, is of two varieties: (1) the *distinct*, when the pustules are separate and well defined; (2) the *confluent*, when they are thick-set, run into each other, and form continuous suppurating surfaces. In this latter variety all the symptoms are aggravated, the glands are affected, the limbs swell, the mucous membranes show the eruption, and there is danger of suffocation from involvement of the larynx. This variety is, therefore, very dangerous, for the severity bears a direct proportion to the extent and suppuration of the pustules.

Mode of Propagation—By contagion. No contagion is so strong, so sure, or operates at so great a distance of time and place. It is probably most infectious when the characteristic odour is perceived, and when the pustules suppurate. Recurrence of the disease is rare.

Symptoms—At first these are similar to those of most other fevers. There is lassitude, chilliness, heat, headache, a *thickly-furred white tongue*, a deep flush upon the face, a feeling of *bruised pain* all over the body, *but especially in the back and loins*, more or less pain or *tenderness at the pit of the stomach*, and sometimes vomiting. On the second and third days there may be transitory rashes of scarlatinal or measly type. These sometimes lead to errors of diagnosis, but their usual distribution, confined to lower abdomen, sides of thorax, axillae, and inner sides of thighs, should prevent mistakes. On about the third day the eruption appears in the form of red spots, or small hard pimples, feeling like *shot in the skin*. It first comes out on the forehead and front of the wrists; then on the neck and breast; then gradually extends over the body.

The eruption being completed, the fever subsides; the pimples begin to fill with fluid matter; this is first watery and transparent (vesicles), then yellowish (pustules); they become *depressed in the centre* ("umbilicated"), and are surrounded by a circular inflamed ring. The eyelids, face, and hands are swollen, and the features sometimes obliterated. A peculiarly disagreeable odour now emanates from the patient, which, once smelt, cannot be forgotten. In about eight or nine days from the first appearance of the eruption, the pustules discharge their contents; secondary fever seats in; scabs then form, which dry up, and, in a strong constitution, fall off in the course of four or five days. There remain purplish spots, which do not fade away before the sixth or eighth week, or indelible depressed scars, which are called *pits* or *pocks*. Discrete variola rarely leaves pocks; confluent variola always does.

Diagnosis—Unlike *Measles* and *Scarlet fever*, the pimples give the sensation to the finger of small show embedded in the skin; the catarrhal symptoms of Measles, and the sore throat of Scarlet fever, are absent. Unlike *Chicken-pox*, the eruption suppurates and the fever is high. Unlike *Enteric fever*, the onset is abrupt.

Danger—The more numerous and confluent the pustules, the grater the danger; the more perfect their maturity on the fourth day, the less the danger. The greatest danger arises from the *secondary fever*, about the ninth to the twelfth day, while the pustules are ripening; for then the fever is likely to return, when the vital strength is already much exhausted. In a confluent case, fatal chest symptoms may arise, or abscesses may from in various parts of the body, or there may be ulceration and opacity of the cornea and loss of sight. Suppressed perspiration, scanty urine, Haematuria, great hoarseness, Convulsions, Delirium, or other complications increase the danger of fatality. Half the deaths occur between the seventh and eleventh days of the eruption. Smallpox is very fatal to young children. Small, dark, and badly ventilated dwellings, poor or scanty food, and want of cleanliness, constitute unfavourable conditions.

Treatment—*Ant.-Tart.* is considered to be the most suitable medicine, and a dose should be given every two or three hours. It may be proceeded by a few doses of *Acon.* at similar intervals, and the two medicines may be administered alternately, if the violence of the fever demand the continuance of the *Acon.* Uncomplicated cases will in all probability yield to this treatment.

Indications for the above and other Remedies

Aconitum—Fever, headache, rapid pulse, etc.

Antimonium Tart.—This remedy should be given as soon as Smallpox is suspected. Spasmodic retching, nausea, and hoarse cough, often very distressing, may be relieved, Convulsions averted, and the severity of the disease greatly modified by it.

Apis.—Considerable *swelling of the face and eyelids.* If the swelling be attended with *hoarseness*, and pain in swallowing, *Apis.* and *Bell.* should be alternated.

Belladonna—Stupor or delirium, *severe headache,* dislike of light, Opthalmia. *Bell.* also tends to retain the eruption upon the surface.

Coffea.—Restlessness and *sleeplessness.*

Comphor—If the eruption suddenly disappear, or suddenly assume a malignant type, with coldness of the skin, difficult breathing, disorder of the brain, etc., one or two drops in a little *tepid* water, or on a small piece of sugar, every ten or fifteen minutes, till the skin becomes warm, and the eruption reappears. The blanket-bath may be had recourse to with much benefit at the same time.

Mercurius Sol. 6.—Ulcerated throat, *Salivation, and Diarrhoea,* with bloody stools; especially during suppuration.

Sulphur—When the disease pursues an irregular course; when the eruption shows a tendency to recede; when the pustules are green, purple or black; during the formation of the pustules; when there is excessive itching; and especially on the decline of the disease, to prevent the usual sequelae, the *tincture of Sulph.* is especially valuable.

Additional Remedies—*Acon.* (inflammation generally); *Apis.* (dropsical swellings); *Ars.* (prostration); *Bell.* (delirium, inflamed throat); *Bry.* (bronchitis); *Carb. Veg.* (gastric disorder with putrescence); *Hyos.* (delirium and restlessness); *Kali Bich.* (bronchitis); *Merc.* (glandular swellings); *Phosph.* (pneumonia); *Rhus. Tox.* (pain in back); *Stram.* (delirium).

Accessories—The patient should be placed in a moderately lighted room, in which there is ample provision made for the uninterrupted admission of fresh air, and the free escape of tainted air. A lighted fire and an open window are almost essential in all seasons. The patient's eyes should be screened from the direct rays of light. He should be kept cool and scrupulously clean, and his sheets and linen frequently changed. His posture in bed should be frequently changed, so as to avoid constant lying on his back or on particular parts; otherwise troublesome bed-sores are apt to be formed. As soon as the eruption is well out, the uncovered parts (face, hands, wrists) may be covered with lint soaked in dilute carbolic acid (1 in 80). This is grateful to the patient and helps considerably to allay the irritation. It is desirable in any case to protect the ripening pimples from the light. As the pimples begin to ripen into pustules. they should be kept moist with olive oil, glycerine and water, or vaseline. The process should be repeated as often as necessary. The hands of the children should always be muffled to prevent them scratching.

Special attention must be paid to the eyes, which should be washed out, and the eyelids carefully cleaned, with weak boracic lotion several times a day. The mouth, throat and nose should also be swabbed out.

Disinfection—All infected clothing and bedding should

be *burned;* or, in default of this, baked or boiled for half an hour at a temperature of 212°. Rooms should be fumigated with burning *Sulphur,* the walls cleansed and divested of their paper, the floors scrubbed and washed with a solution of Chloride of Zinc, and walls and ceiling lime-washed; afterwards the doors and windows kept open for several days. (See Preventive Measures, chapter II, page 09).

Diet—During the presence of the primary and secondary fever, the diet should be chiefly milk and soda-water, gruel, plain, or simple yolks of eggs beaten up with cold milk, grapes, oranges, cooked fruits, etc. For drink, cold water, with or without the addition of raspberry-vinegar or currant-jelly; toast-water, barley-water, lemonade, etc. Ordinary simple and *nutritious* diet may be taken in the absence of fever. But as the mucous membrane as well as the skin is affected, care must be taken not to irritate it.

Preventive during an Epidemic—*Vaccination* (see next Section); tincture of *Sulphur,* administered once or twice daily for several days, and *fresh air.* Too much importance cannot be attached to the dilution and dispersion of the Smallpox poison by free ventilation and disinfectants, which operate as preventive for the unaffected, and improve the condition of patients suffering from the disease. The spread of an epidemic of Smallpox is just in proportion to the overcrowded and insanitary condition of the places in which it occurs.

VACCINATION—COW-POX

This disease is not natural to man, but to the cow. It is similar to Smallpox; and when artificially introduced into the human system is as nearly as possible without being absolutely, protective against Smallpox.

During the last fifty years, since its general use, it has probably saved more human lives (to say nothing of disfigurement, loss of sight, etc.) than all other remedies put together. It has fallen into disrepute in some quarters on account of the troublesome affections that have occasionally followed it. These, however, bear but a very small proportion to the number of cases in which no secondary effects appeared, and are not to be mentioned in comparison with the loathsomeness and fatality of Smallpox. Without doubt, in a few cases the communication of some other disorder has accompanied Vaccination, through the carelessness or ignorance of the vaccinator. But it is also unquestionable that in a great many cases it has only been the occasion, not the cause, of another disorder. Anything which sets up a temporary febrile condition may develop a latent disease; and as Vaccination is usually among the first dirturbers of the system, it has borne the discredit of causing what it only stimulated. The occurance of troublesome consequences only show that the vaccine should be administered by the careful and skilful practitioner under aseptic conditions.

Vaccination is advisable during the first three months of infancy, before dentition disturbs the system. In the event of parents having a "conscientious objection" to vaccination, a certificate of exemption may be obtained from a magistrate, or if the child suffers from any disease which renders Vaccination undesirable, a medical certificate may be obtained to that effect. Three precautions should be observed: (1) The *lymph* should never be taken from another child, as was done in a past generation, but should be freshly obtained from some reliable source, such as the Lister Institute in London. (2) A *clean lancet* or *needle* should be employed. (3) The lymph should be dabbed on two or three places on one arm or leg, and the places should be sacrified through the lymph until the blood is just seen.

Symptoms—When the operation is successful a slight rosy elevation may be seen and felt on the second day, and a small red pimple is formed on the third day, while the temperature rises slightly. On the fifth day a vesicle forms, which reaches its maximum size on the eighth day, being then distended with limpid fluid and distinctly "umbilicated." By the tenth day the fluid is purulent. By the fourteenth day the pustule has become a brownish scab, which about the twenty-first day falls off, leaving a circular, depressed, permanent scar.

The constitutional disturbance is usually not great. From the third to the ninth days a little fever and restlessness may show themselves, and sometimes swelling in the armpit. Medical treatment is seldom necessary. Should there be much inflammatory redness and swelling, a few doses of *Aconite or Belladonna* will relieve the patient. The latter remedy is curative of *erysipelatous* complications. Care should be taken to protect the arms from friction, that the sores may not be irritated, and the scabs not torn off. Occasionally a poultice is necessary if inflammation or suppuration is excessive. About the eighth day, as the disorder declines, a dose of *Sulphur*, morning and night, for a few days, may prevent possible unpleasant sequels.

Re-vaccination—Although it is impossible to tell how long the protective virtue of vaccine lasts, it may be well if Vaccination were repeated at puberty. In like manner adults may secure immunity, if Smallpox become epidemic, by being vaccinated again. Carefully recorded observations and statistics show that well-vaccinated persons are almost wholly secure against infection.

CHICKEN-POX

This is an eruption almost peculiar to infants and young

children, and bears some resemblance to Smallpox, for which it may be mistaken. It spreads by contagion.

Symptoms—On the second day of a slight fever the eruption appears. The pimples rapidly become pustular, and in three or four days from their appearance dry up, forming scabs, which fall off in six or seven days without leaving permanent scars. The eruption comes out irregularly, and in successive crops, so that while some of the pustules are disappearing, others may be forming.

It differs from Smallpox in the slighter fever which attends it; in the earlier appearance of the eruption; in the absence of an inflammatory ring around the spots in the first stage in the vesicular character of the eruption, the spots of which become filled with a watery fluid about the second or third day, which is converted into yellow matter; and in the rapid course of the complaint.

Treatment—In may cases little medicine will be needed; but in the early state, *Acon.* every three hours will modify any fever that may be present. Afterwards *Rhus* should be given every three or four hours until convalescence sets in.

Indications for these and other Remedies

Aconitum—Hot skin, thirst, and other febrile symptoms.

Ant.-Tart.—Convulsions.

Apis.—Excessive itching of the skin, or puffy swelling of the eyelids.

Belladonna—For severe headache and any disturbance of the brain.

Mercurius Sol. 6—If suppuration takes place in any of the pimples.

Rhus Tox.—This is the best remedy for the disease, and unless any of the other remedies are strongly indicated, should be given as soon as possible.

Accessories—Attention to diet as in simple fever, especially if the digestive organs are impaired. Milk diet is best. Exposure to cold should be avoided, especially in cold weather, but the room should be kept well ventilated. The child should be prevented from scratching the skin when the scales are formed.

SIMPLE FEVER (Febricula)

This not now believed to be a distinct disease. In some cases it may be *Influenza*, but Influenza is not common in children. Probably many cases called febricula or "chill" are *rheumatic*, representing a quite brief invasion of the microbe of Rheumatism (see "Rheumatism" of Children," page 67). In many cases there is a slight soreness of the throat, suggestive of a *tonsillar* infection. In some children *Constipation* causes a slight fever, cut short when the bowels act freely. In quite a number of children it is due to *bacilluria* or an infection of the bladder with *bacillus coli* (see "Bacilluria," page 183). There is also a classes of febricula of obscure alimentary origin, sometimes called "food-fever" or "bilious attacks"; these often recur more or less periodically (see "Chronic Vomiting," page 144, and "Appendicitis," page 152).

Treatment—If the symptoms, as is often the case, are sudden feeling of chilliness followed by, or perhaps alternating with, flushes of heat, dry skin, full quick pulse, coated tongue, thirst, highly-coloured and scanty urine, headache, pain in loins, slight sore throat, loss of appetite— the symptoms of what is often called a "chill," a Camphor pilule every twenty minutes for three times may be all that is necessary; but if that stage has passed, *Acon.* should be given at once, and repeated every hour, two hours, or three hours, according to the violence of the symptoms.

Indications for the above and
other Remedies

Aconitum—Chills, followed by great heat and dryness of skin; dry mouth, lips, and tongue; thirst; full, hard, and frequent pulse; hurried breathing, and scanty urine.

Arsenicum—In some protracted cases, where there is great prostration with feeble pulse.

Belladonna—When there is intense headache, flushing of the face, congestion of the eyes, and great dread of light and noise.

Bryonia—Severe muscular pains; painful cough; oppressed breathing.

Camphor—Severe chills, with lassitude.

Accessories—Quiet, repose in bed. Light bed coverings. The warm bath (see page 15), the hot foot bath, or the wet-pack. Water should be the principal beverage, in small repeated draughts; it encourages perspiration, promotes the beneficial action of the bath or pack, and lessens thirst. As the fever declines, milk diet should precede more substantial food.

ENTERIC FEVER—TYPHOID FEVER

Definition—Formerly always known as Typhoid fever, now more accurately called Enteric fever, it is a general infection, with local manifestations in the "solitary glands" and Peyer's patches of the intestine.

Causation—The real cause is the *Bacillus typhosus* of Eberth, which is conveyed to a very small extent by contagion or transmission through the air, but chiefly by contaminated *water* and *food*, especially *milk*, sometimes *oysters*. The recent great improvements in sanitation have had their reward in a great diminution of Enteric fever. But a factor in the spread of the disease, always doubtless existing but not formerly recognized, has recently been brought to light—the typhoid "carrier." Persons not actually suffering from Enteric, though they may have had it, may still "carry" the germs and thus be a source of infection— the milk, e.g., may thus get infected at dairies.

Predisposing causes are (*a*) youth. It is a disease especially of the second and third decades of life. "It is not very infrequent in childhood, but infants are rarely attacked" (Osler). (*b*) Season of year. It is a disease of autumn, especially after a long period of hot dry weather.

Symptoms—Enteric fever is usually insidious in its invasion, the early symptoms being those of indigestion, languor, poor appetite, constipation, pain in the head, occasionally nose-bleeding, sleeplessness, dull wandering mind, and often delirium at night. The patient complains of much weakness, thirst, and has a dry, red-coated, or cracked tongue. The early pulse is not so fast as would be expected from the fever, but later is becomes quick and feeble, the skin is hot, and a bright circumscribed flush appears on the cheek. Enlargement of the abdomen and Diarrhoea take place, with tenderness on the right side, below the level of the navel (the right iliac region), and a gurgling feeling is produced there on pressure ; there is also increased dullness over the spleen from its enlargement. *The diarrhoeic discharges* are of *light ochre* colour, copious, liquid (the "pea-soup" stool), and in advanced stages of the disease often contain altered blood. Often, however, there is constipation and not diarrhoea.

The *eruption* appears after about the seventh day, and consists of a few rose-coloured dots, which fade away for a moment on pressure. The little spots appears in children chiefly on the abdomen, lower thorax, and back. In a few days each spot disappears, to be succeeded by others.

F-5

The *temperature* mounts gradually ("staircase" temperature), rising 2° every night and falling 1° every morning for the first week.

Just as during the increase of the disease the temperature *gradually* rises, so in recovery the decline in the temperature is *gradual*, not sudden as it is in *Typhus*.

A *persistent* temperature of 104°, after end of the second week, is unfavourable, as is also persistent acceleration of the pulse.

Left to themselves, mild cases are over in twentyone days, but severe ones may last four or five weeks, or even much longer.

Diagnosis—Enteric fever is sometimes mistaken for other diseases, especially for Pulmonary Phthisis. In Phthisis, cough and dyspnoea appear earlier and are more severe than in Enteric fever. There are also present the stethoscopic signs of tubercle in the former disease. The typhoid rash and enlargement of the spleen are absent from the consumptive patient. Enteric fever may be mistaken for Typhus, but Typhus is practically extinct in this country. The laboratory test, known as the Widal test, available after the first week of the disease, if positive is diagnostic of Enteric; as is also the discovery of the *Bac. typhosus* in the stools.

Danger—Perforation of the bowel and fatal haemorrhage are possibilities, but they are not common in children. Danger may also arise from lung complications—Pneumonia, Bronchitis, or Pleurisy; or the fever may subsequently call into activity latent germs of tubercle.

Treatment—Administered in the early stage, before diarrhoea has set in, *Baptisia* unquestionably modifies the symptoms, and even cuts short an attack. In the absence of complications we prolong its use until convalescence is established. When there is profuse diarrhoea *Arsenicum* will probably be required.

Indications for the above and
other Remedies

Arsenicum—In a late stage of the disease when there is a good deal of purging of thin feculent matter of a *light-ochre* colour, with or without blood.

Baptisia—Pain in the forehead, flushed face, sleeplessness, slight nocturnal delirium, thirst, thinly white coated tongue, frequent soft pulse, and heat of skin.

Bryonia—stands next to *Baptisia* in its relation to the disease. It is indicated by the following symptoms: Headache, flushed face, bitter taste in the mouth, heat of skin, and pains in the limbs.

Muriatic Acid—In putrid sore throat, great depression.

Additional Remedies—*Bell.* (when the brain is involved): *Carbo V.* (offensive and putrid exhalations and excretions); *China* (debility during convalescence); *Ferrum* (as for *China*); *Hyos.* (restlessness); *Merc.* (copious perspirations); *Phosph.* (pneumonia); *Phosph.-Ac* (debility with much perspiration); *Sulph.* (in convalescence).

Secondary Diseases—If any troublesome affections arise during convalescence, reference must be made to other parts of this work. We may, however, suggest *Iod., Bry.,* or *Phos.,* for disorders of the chest; *Carbo V., Ign., Merc.,* or *Nux V.,* for indigestion; *Bell., Hyos., Opi., Zinc.,* or *Rhus,* for disorders of the brain. *Deafness* usually disappears with the return of strength, which may be promoted by *China, Phos.-Ac.,* or *Sulph. China* also moderates hunger, and facilitates the repair necessitated by waste of the fluids of the body. *Sulph.* aids recuperative efforts.

Accessories—As in Smallpox and Scarlet fever, the ventilation of the apartment should be as thorough as open doors and windows and a good fire can make it, while the patient should be protected from draught and kept comfortably warm by additional blankets. Light and sound should be subdued. All unnecessary furniture, and every vessel that is not clean, should be removed. Vessels to receive the excretions should be ready prepared with some disinfectant freely employed, and afterwards removed immediately. A second bed or couch, to which the patient could be removed, affords relief and change of air immediately around his body.

But the recumbent posture must be maintained, even during early convalescence. Any violent or sudden movement might occasion a relapse. The linen, including blankets, should be frequently changed. The mouth may be often wiped out with a soft towel, wetted in the water which contains a little Condy's fluid, to remove the *sordes* which gather there in low forms of fever. Frequent sponging with tepid or cold water or *vinegar and water,* drying quickly with a soft towel, is very refreshing and healthful. The body may be sponged piecemeal to avoid fatigue. Spots subject to pressure like the lower part of the back should be carefully washed with methylated spirit, then carefully dried and dusted with a mixture of starch powder and zinc oxide, to prevent the formation of bed-sores. An air-ring or an air-bed may be also used for the same purpose. Where a bed-sore has formed, it should be kept scrupulously clean and calendula ointment used as a dressing.

Diet—At the commencement of the fever, pure water, toast-and-water, gum-water sweetened (1oz. gum arabic, ½ oz. loaf sugar, to one pint of hot water), soda-water, or lemonade is nearly all that will be required. Cold water lowers the temperature of the body, and aids the medical treatment. On account of the dry and shrivelled state of the tongue, the patient is often unable to relish or swallow any food. To lubricate the mucous membranes and stimulate the savilary glands, a little lemon-juice and water may be given a few minutes before the food. Everything taken into the stomach should be fluid or semifluid, until convalescence is established. Milk, arrowroot made with milk, blancmange of isinglass, cornflour, or ground rice, yolk of egg betan up with milk, white of egg in water ("albumen water"), cold beef-tea, and slightly thickened broths, are nutritious. Nourishment should be given with strict regularity, and frequently. If milk is being given, the stools should be inspected for curds; if curds are found, diminish the amount of milk. If there is diarrhoea, animal broths and beef-tea are liable to aggravate it. During convalescence, food should only be allowed in great moderation, and never to the capacity of the appetite till the tongue is clean and moist, and the pulse and skin normal. Solids given too early have caused relapse. Change of air, when the child is able to walk, will prove serviceable in establishing his health.

DIPHTHERIA

Definition—A contagious febrile disease in which there is exudation of lymph on the lining of the throat, especially the tonsils, soft palate, and upper part of the air-passages, attended with much general prostration, from blood-poisoning; the throat symptoms being secondary to the blood contamination. It is most important to distinctly recognize the fact that Diphtheria is a constitutional disease; that the constitutional disturbance are the *primary* symptoms, and not *secondary* to the physical changes about the throat; and that, therefore, efforts should be made to deal with the whole systemic mischief, rather than to concentrate the attention on the tangible local effects.

Causes—The real or microbic cause of Diphtheria is the *Klebs-Loeffler bacillus*. The infection is carried from person to person, mainly amongst the young, but fairly often also amongst adults. The virus, which is carried mainly from the membranous exudates and discharges, whether of throat or nose, adheres persistently to walls and furniture, and is apt to attack several members of the same family. Autumn is the diphtheria season. This is one of the diseases communicated by healthy "carriers" who are either convalescent from the disease or have never had it. Enlarged tonsils and a general unhealthy condition of the mucous membrane of the mouth and throat are probably predisposing causes.

Symptoms—The early symptoms are those of fever, the temperature not usually rising above 101° or 102°, with redness and soreness of the throat. Then a patchy greyish-white exudation (the "membrane") appears on the tonsils and gradually spreads over the soft palate and uvula, and it may be, on to the pharynx. The glands in the neck are swollen and there is greater or less dysphagia (pain on swallowing).

In severe cases the local lesions progress, the membrane extends downwards into the larynx and upwards into the nose, there is severe sloughing and great fetor, the glands become greatly enlarged, the temperature sinks, the pulse becomes weak and rapid, there may be uncontrolable vomiting and partial or complete suppression of urine, the patient is of an ashy pallor and collapse threatens. This condition, which is one of profound systemic toxaemia, comes on about the eleventh day. Where the larynx is involved, there may be violent attacks of dyspnoea, ending finally in suffocation or coma.

Diagnosis—For diagnosis from *Croup,* page 113. The main diagnostic difficulty connected with Diphtheria is to distinguish it from other forms of sore throat. The chief practical difficulty is to distinguish a diphtheritic exudation from that seen in Follicular Tonsillitis (where there are multiple yellowish-white spots at the orifices of the tonsillar crypts). The chief diagnostic points are as follows:— the higher temperatures are seen in Follicular Tonsillitis, the lower in

Diphtheria; there is greater prostration and depression in diphtheria; albuminuria and loss of knee-jerks point to Diphtheria; removal of the exudation with a wool-tipped probe is difficult in Diphtheria owing to the adherence of the membrane, and is apt to be attended with bleeding. If there is any doubt as to the nature of an exudation on the tonsils or fauces, a swab should be taken and sent to a laboratory.

Sequelae—The most important is *Paralysis*, coming on usually in the second or third week of convalescence, due to a peripheral neuritis. The chief palsies are (*a*) of the *palate*, causing the patient on attempting to swallow his food to bring it back through the nose, (*b*) of the *eye-muscles*, causing squint or dropping (ptosis) of the upper eyelid, (*c*) a paralysis of the *heart muscle*, causing, it may be, a great slowing of the pulse or even sudden syncope, which may be fatal.

Treatment—Alloathic mortality has undoubtedly been greatly reduced by the adoption of the *antitoxin* treatment. Homoeopaths are divided as to whether they should use antitoxin or not. A case treated with homoeopathic remedies from the very outset will probably never need anything else. But medical advice may not be sought until the case has advanced well beyond the initial state; and besides, causes of very exceptional virulence may at any time crop up which task our therapeutic resources to the utmost. It is a question, then, under these circumstances whether it is not wise and right to use antitoxin. It should be remembered that antitoxin is neither allopathic nor homoeopathic. The treatment consists in neutralizing a poison and so rendering it inert, much as Condy's fluid (permanganate of potash) neutralizes opium when it has been taken poisonously into the stomach. There is no reason at all why homoeopathic remedies should not be administered concurrently with the injection of antitoxin. 2,000 to 4,000 units for a mild case, increased up to 10,000 or 15,000 for more severe cases, may be injected (with strict regard to asepsis) under the skin of the lower abdomen. A patient known to suffer from Asthma or to have had an antitoxin injection on a former occasion ought probably *not* to be injected (Good all).

Treatment—*Bell.* should be given at once. In mild cases this medicine may be sufficient, given a dose every two hours. If no improvement follows its action in about forty-eight hours, *Merc.-Cyan.* should be administered every three hours. *Mur.-Ac* may afterwards be had recourse to if the *Merc.-Cyan.* fail to produce any satisfactory result.

Indications for the above and other Remedies

Ammon.-Carb.—Burning sensation in the throat, and when there is great physical and mental prostration, especially in the last stage.

Arsenicum—Cold, clammy sweats, frequent, small pulse, Diarrhoea, great thirst, and much prostration.

Belladonna—Throat red and swollen, with white patches studded over it, dryness of the throat, thirst, etc.

Gelseminum—For resulting paralysis.

Iodium—When the affection has spread to the wind-pipe, and produces symptoms of Croup.

Kali Bichrom—When the disease extends into the nostrils this medicine may be selected.

Kali Permangan—In some of the worst cases with intense foetor of the breath this medicine appears to have acted beneficially.

Merc.-Bin.—Swelling and deep-red appearance of the throat, with specks of exudation, and excessive foetid secretion.

Merc.-Cyan.—For pronounced Diphtheria; great depression; formation of false membranes.

Mur.-Ac.—Putrid state of throat, dry parched tongue, great weakness, relaxes bowels, etc.

Additional Remedies—*China* and *Helonias* (debility of convalescence); *Con.* and *Dig.* (enfeebled heart); *Phyto.* and *Phosph.* (hoarseness).

Local Treatment—At the outset of the disease hot fomentations or poultices should be applied around the throat. Where the child will permit it, the throat and nose may be flushed out frequently with warm solution of boracic acid. Alternatively, he may inhale over a jug of boiling water in which is a teaspoonful of carbolic acid. When the larynx is involved, a steam tent should be rigged up over the bed.

Where dyspnoea becomes extreme from laryngeal obstruction, tracheotomy must be resorted to.

During convalescence the patient should "hasten slowly." Any signs of Paralysis are a signal for putting the convalescent to bed for a protracted season. A change of air is highly desirable.

Warm Baths—These are valuable accessories in the early stage. The skin is hot and dry, the urine is often suppressed. the bowels confined, and thus the poison is retained in the system. Warm baths, and drinking freely of cold water, often restore the functions of the skin, the bladder and bowels.

Diet, etc.—The strength of the patient must be sustained, from the very commencement of the disease, by nourishment, and he must be urged to swallow it in spite of the pain which it occasions. Eggs beaten up in milk, with sugar; beef-tea slightly thickened with rice or pearl-barley; arrowroot or sago.

If vomiting occur, sucking small pieces of ice will tend to allay it. Ice also affords comfort to the patient, and favours the action of the kidneys.

Preventive Measures—The cesspool should be emptied, and if too small or defective, new ones built. The house,

water-closets, and local drainage should be thoroughly
examined, and imperfections rectified; also, if necessary,
chloride of zinc or of lime constantly kept therein, and thrown
down the drains. All dust-holes and accumulations of refuse
should be cleared away; a plentiful supply of water kept in the
house, and every room regularly well-cleaned, whitewashed,
and thoroughly ventilated.

WHOOPING-COUGH (Pertussis)

Definition—A paroxysmal cough, chiefly affecting
infancy and childhood; consisting of violent, spasmodic fits
of coughing, ending in prolonged, shrill, crowing
inspirations, and the vomiting of thick, glairy mucus.

Whooping-cough is both epidemic and contagious.
Infants under three years of age are specially liable to it; it is
rare after ten. The younger the infant the more dangerous
the disease. It frequently occurs as an epidemic about the
same time as Measles, and though this may be at any time
of the year, these disorders are specially prevalent in spring
and autumn. The duration of the disorder varies from two
or three weeks to many months. This depends very much on
the temperament and constitution of the child. But the
duration of the disease may be much abridged by
homoeopathic treatment.

Cause and Mode of Spreading—The disease is doubtless
of microbic origin, but it is not certain what the microbe is.
The disease is apt to be epidemic and is mainly
communicated from person to person. It often follows or
precedes Measles and Scarlet fever.

Symptoms—Whooping-cough usually commences as a
Catarrh, with cough, which returns in fits at intervals. In
about a week the cough recurs at shorter intervals, in

paroxysms of extreme severity, the child turning red or almost black in the face, and appears as if choking, during which the lungs are emptied of air to the last degree, and then a long, sonorous inspiration, taken to refill them, constitutes the "whoop."

This "whoop" is the signal of the child's safety, for where suffocation does take place it is before the crowing inspiration has been made. The attacks recur every two or three hours, or, in severe cases, oftener, and sometimes blood escapes from the nose, mouth, and even from the ears. The successive fits pass off with the expectoration of glairy, ropy mucus, and sometimes with Vomiting. Between the attacks there is such freedom from pain and ease of breathing that the child is lively and cheerful.

Weakness and loss of flesh are, however, occasioned by the repeated ejection of food from the stomach, and by the terror with which the child anticipates the attacks. The cough is generally worse at night, so that a decline of nocturnal attacks is a favourable symptom. But it may be brought back with all its severity by exposure to cold, by improper food, and by want of proper nursing during the period of convalescence. In any case it is rarely fatal, though danger is greater during the colder seasons of the year, and in young infants and delicate children.

Complications—Whooping-cough may be complicated by haemorrhages under the skin, especially of the face, and by haemoptysis. Convulsions are not very rare. The most important complications are Bronchitis (practically always present more or less), Broncho-Pneumonia (the most fatal of all), which often becomes tuberculous, Lymphadenitis of the bronchial glands, Emphysema, and Cardiac Dilatation. There may also be wasting and anaemia. These complications and sequelae made Whooping-cough a very fatal disease under non-homoeopathic treatment.

Diagnosis—If the "whoop" is not actually heard, the diagnosis may be difficult. The points that help are the paroxysmal character of the cough, the occurrence of Vomiting, the puffiness of the eyes, and the presence of a sublingual ulcer (due to protrusion of the tongue during cough and the catching of the *frenum* of the tongue against the lower incisor teeth). All paroxysmal cough is not Whooping-cough. The disease may be simulated by the cough caused by enlarged bronchial glands. A history of tubercle or of a former attack of Whooping-cough (which is not likely to be repeated but is very likely to be followed by enlarged bronchial glands) would point to Bronchial Lymphadenitis. The best way to establish such a diagnosis would be to examine the chest with the X-rays.

Treatment—In the early state the symptoms are usually those of common cold, and point to *Acon.* and then to *Ipecac.*, which medicines may be given alternately, or otherwise, as the case may demand. When the spasmodic and peculiarly characteristic "whoop" is decided, *Drosera* should be administered—a dose every three hours.

Indications for the above and other Remedies

Aconitum—Febrile symptoms, dry cough, burning pain in larynx.

Belladonna—Dry cough, spasmodic contraction of larynx, sore throat, flushed face, suffused eyes, convulsions.

Cuprum—Paroxysms attended with threatened suffocation, Vomiting, rattling noise in bronchial tubes, Convulsions.

Drosera—Similar to *Cuprum*, but without Convulsions.

Ipecacuanha—Dry cough; Vomiting, especially in the

early state of the disease.

Additional Remedies—*Ant.-Tart.* (Bronchitis, with much sputa); *Byr.* (Pleuritis); *Carbol.-Ac.* (premonitory Catarrh); *Coral.-Rub.* (fully developed symptoms, return of cough after it has apperantly left the patient); *Cina* (Cough, with gastric derangement, Worms); *Dulcam.* (aggravated by damp); *Kali Bich.* (Bronchitis, with stringy mucus); *Phosph.* (Pneumonia). *Ammon.-Brom.*—Drs. Harley and Gibbs regard this remedy as almost specific, and many cures by it are reported.

Accessories—In warm, fine weather the patient may take exercise in the open air during portions of each day; indeed, a reasonable degree of exposure to open air, in the absence of unfavourable conditions, is one of the most essential aids towards recovery. But damp and draughts should be strictly avoided, as the skin is generally relaxed, sensitive to cold, and after a paroxysm bathed in perspiration. Warm clothing is therefore necessary. Fits of anger add to the frequency and violence of the paroxysms. Infants must be watched day and night, taken up as soon as a fit comes on, and placed in a favourable posture. "Balcony" treatment, or its equivalent, is of the utmost value, and is only contra-indicated by strong winds and fog. In obstinate cases, *change of air,* if only at a short distance, often proves a great utility.

Another means of relief is to rub the chest and back of the little sufferer with oil for a few minutes every morning and night. Spinal friction is also of service.

Diet—Light digestible food only, in moderate quantities, frequently given; in the convulsive stage it should be highly nutritious and if there is much vomiting, it should be given immediately after a paroxysm. Toast-and-water, barley-water, or gum-water are grateful and soothing; but a too exclusive slop-diet often aggravates the vomiting. Cod-liver oil should be given in convalescence.

MUMPS (Parotitis)

Definition—Inflammatory swelling of the salivary (parotid) glands beneath and in front of the ear, frequently with pain, soreness, and difficulty in moving the jaws. The glands sometimes attain a very large size; the enlargement generally commences on one side, and as it diminishes shows itself on the other side.

Causes—A specific germ of uncertain identity, communicated by direct contact. It often occurs as an epidemic, particularly in cold, damp weather; is more incident to children after the fifth year than to adults; and only occasionally attacks the same person twice. It is very infectious; children take it from their playmates and school fellows.

Symptoms—At first there is a feeling of stiffness and soreness on moving the jaw, and the child complains of the discomfort of eating; indeed, the pain caused by eating or even drinking is sometimes agonizing. The swelling first appears in the hollow under one ear and spreads downwards in the neck and forwards on to the face; two or three days later the parotid gland on the opposite side of the face begins to swell. The glands continue to be sore and painful, with more or less fever and headache, for about a week. There is little danger, but there are one or two unfortunate possible complications, such as *Deafness*, *Orchitis* (inflammation of the testicles—this, however, seldom occurs before puberty), and *Pancreatitis* (severe epigastric pain, vomiting, and collapse).

Treatment—Give *Acon.* every two or three hours for three or four times, then *Merc.-Sol.* 6 every three hours.

Indications for the above and other Remedies.

Aconitum—Pain and fever.

Belladonna—Pain, erysipelatous redness of the skin, tendency to meatastasis of the brain.

Mercurius Sol.—Foul tongue, increased flow of saliva.

Pulsatilla—When metastasis takes place to the testicles or mammae.

Accessory Means—The child should be kept in a warm room, but not confined to bed. The parts may be fomented with hot water several times a day, and in the intervals covered with a flannel bandage. The patient should be protected from cold, damp, and excitement. In this disease, as also in Quinsy, semi-liquid food is swallowed with much less suffering that either liquid or solid food, and hence should be chiefly used.

Chapter II

CONSTITUTIONAL DISEASES

RHEUMATISM OF CHILDREN

Rheumatism is a very common disease in children, and owing in particular to its effect upon the heart, it is productive of a great deal of ill-health, chronic invalidism, and premature death. The adult type of acute Articular Rheumatism (Rheumatic fever) is seldom seen in children. Rather is the condition subacute, and indeed often afebrile. Whereas in adults the force of the disease expends itself on the joints, in children there is comparatively little of rheumatic pain, and when present it is not severe, but the disease takes terrible toll of the heart and nervous system.

Definition—A microbic infection constitutionally causing a low range of fever and an often profound anaemia and locally affecting the joints, the fibrous and muscular tissues, the throat, the tissues of the heart, and the cortex of the brain.

Causation—The real cause is almost certainly a microorganism, which probably in most cases gets access into the body through the tonsils. Hence the Tonsillitis, which is an early manifestation often repeated through the course of the disease. Exciting causes are chill and damp and insufficiency of warm clothing. Low-lying soil which keeps the damp and garments improperly "aired"—or garments sat in when they are damp, all make a heavy contribution to the sum-total of Rheumatism. The influence of food as a causative factor is probably negligible. The "acidity" of Rheumatism is not due to uric acid, as is so commonly supposed, but rather to *latic acid*, manufactured in the muscles through the activity of the specific microbe.

Symptoms—The main manifestations of Rheumatism in children are Tonsillitis, slight and fugitive pains in joints and muscles (favourite sites are the back of the knee and the heel), nodules on the exposed bony surfaces and prominences (e.g. elbow, ulna, wrist, vertebrae), Carditis (inflammation of the heart—Peri-, Myo-, and Endo-carditis), Chorea (St. Vitus's Dance (see page 95), minor nervous symptoms (e.g. night-terrors, incontinence of urine, teeth-griding, etc.), erythematous rashes, Rheumatic Anaemia, and the symptoms of Rheumatic Carditis. In this last-named condition there is usually some fever, though it may be slight, and there are vague and inconstant physical signs (enlargement of the heart, murmurs, etc.), but often an increase in the pulse rate is the chief and most reliable guide to the condition. In a rheumatic child, perhaps suffering from some of the other troubles of Rheumatism, an increase of pulse-rate, not otherwise accounted for, signifies that the heart has been attacked. Other suspicious signs are restlessness, pallor, and anaemia. The appearance of "rheumatic nodules" nearly always means that the heart has been involved. Pericarditis alone of the cardiac affections always has marked physical signs—considerable enlargement of the heart's area and the typical to-and-fro rub heard over some part of the heart.

Treatment—*Bry.*, *Rhus Tox.*, and *Merc.-Sol.* are given for the rheumatic pains and Tonsillitis.

Spigelia, *Ars.-Iod.*, *Kalmia*, and *Cactus* are given for the rheumatic heart. For the constitutional condition, the chronic enlargement of the tonsils, and the anaemia, *Calc.-Phos.* is often of the greatest service.

Indications for the above and other Remedies

Aconitum—Pain and fever. Suitable at outset of Rheumatic fever. Often well given in alternation with *Bryonia*.

Arsenicum—Acute Rheumatism with Pericarditis and effusion.

Arsen.-Iod.—Rheumatic Carditis.

Bryonia—Heat and swelling of joints. All pain worse by movement.

Cactus—Rheumatic Carditis.

Calc.-Phos.—Enlarged tonsils. Adenoids. Flatulence and acidity. Chalky pallor. Stiffness, pain, and chilliness, worse from change of weather.

Cimicifuga—Muscular Rheumatism, especially in back and neck. Chorea.

Colchicum—Shifting Rheumatism, worse at night and hot weather. Dysenteric stools. Great nausea from smell of cooking food. Heart trouble, especially Pericarditis.

Dulcamara—Rheumatism from damp and wet, worse by every cold change. Accompanied by Diarrhoea from damp cold weather.

Kalmia—Shifting Rheumatism, Rheumatic iritis. Weak, slow pulse and palpitation.

Pulsatilla—Rheumatic synovitis. Rapidly shifting Rheumatism. Dyspepsia with aversion to fat. Better from cold and in open air. Anaemic. Female remedy.

Rhododendon—Rheumatic pains and swellings, worse at rest. Worst *before* a storm; better after it breaks.

Rhus Tox.—Pain in muscles, tendons, and ligaments; worse at night and in damp cold weather; better from movement.

Ruta—Pain deeply situated, in bones and periosteum, especially of wrist.

Spigelia—Rheumatic headache of forehead and temple, especially on left side. Rheumatism of eye. Rheumatic Carditis—cutting pain in heart and shortness of breath.

Accessory Treatment—Something may be done to prevent Rheumatism, by clothing children properly, particularly the legs and feet, and by seeing that they do not sit in damp clothes. The soundness of the boots should specially be attended do. The tonsils, as a main avenue of infection should be attended to (see *Tonsils and Adenoids,* page 131). The digestion should be attended to, as children are better without much meat; they should certainly not have it more than once a day, and it is well to vary it with fish and eggs.

As regards the actual treatment of Rheumatism, certain rules must be regarded like the laws of the Medes and Persians. The patient must wear wool or flannel next to the skin day and night, summer and winter (in varying thickness). Bathing is good, but may easily be too cold. It the child does not "react" after a cold bath, is blue, chilly, or miserable, the bath must be given up. Rheumatic pains, however slight, are to be treated by putting the child to bed until the pains have passed off. After an attack of acute Rheumatism the child should be kept at rest for several weeks. The object of this is to prevent Rheumatic Carditis. Rest is also the supreme necessity when Rheumatic Carditis has actually supervened. For the treatment of Chorea, see page 95.

RICKETS (Rachitis)

Definition—A constitutional disease characterized by *bony changes* (thickening in some parts, as e.g. at the lower end of the leg and arm bones; softening in other parts owing to the deficiency of mineral phosphates, with resulting deformities), by *catarrhs* (of bronchial tubes, producing Bronchitis; of the bowel, producing Diarrhoea and flatulence), and by *nervous manifestations* (*Convulsions*, see page 85; and *Laryngismus Stridulus*, see page 88).

Symptoms—When a child reaches the tenth month without any appearance of a tooth, or if at two years old he is unable to walk, Rickets may be strongly suspected. A prominent symptom of this disease is *profuse perspiration* of the head, neck, and upper portion of the trunk immediately the child falls asleep, the perspiration standing upon the forehead in beads, or making the pillow wet. The patient desires to lie cool, and kicks off the bed-clothes, both in summer and winter. The child is late in walking, the bones of the leg are curved, and the joint-ends enlarged, especially of the wrists and ankles. The fontanelles are late in closing; the head becomes flat and more square than natural, and the little patient desires to lie still and be undisturbed by playthings or company. The appetite is often voracious and the food passes rapidly, and almost unchanged, through the intestinal canal; there is much straining, and the stools are of variable consistency, and often very loose and offensive. Much generation of gas causes "pot-belly." The flesh is flabby, and there is much muscular weakness and laxity of ligaments; the child is drowsy in the daytime, but restless and uneasy in the night.

In severe cases not merely the leg-bones, but also the spine and pelvis, lose their proper shape; the teeth fall out or soon decay, and the first and second teeth are generally delayed. The chest also become narrow and prominent.

Diagnosis—Rickets may be confounded with Hydro-cephalus; but in the former disease the *fontanelles* (unclosed spaces in the skull of infants) are depressed, while in the latter they are elevated, and often communicate a sensation of pulsation to the hand. The head in Rickets is flat on the top; the head in Hydrocephalus is globular. The distinction between the back in Rickets and the back in Pott's disease or tuberculous disease of the spine (*angular* curvature, as distinct from *lateral* curvature) is that the prominence in Rickets straightens out at once if the child is held up by the armpits; this is not the case in Pott's disease.

Causes—Insanitary surroundings, overcrowding, want of air and especially of sunshine, and defective dietary—often an excess of some starchy proprietary food with deficiency of animal fat and protein (nitrogenous food).

Consequences—These include all kinds of deformities, *bow-legs, pigeon-breast, curvature of the spine, deformed pelvis* (and, in females, consequent *difficult* and *dangerous* labours), and *compression of the internal organs*. If treated early, however, this disease is very remediable, little or no deformity resulting.

Treatment—If commenced early, the best results, with little or no deformity, may be expected. The disease has no definite course to run and at any point the degenerative process may be stayed, a nutritive process initiated, the normal functions restored, and the growth of the child renewed. The medicines in most repute are—*Phosph.-Acid, Silicea, Phosph., Calc.-Carb.* and *Calc.-Phos.*

Indications for the above and other Remedies

Calc.-Carb—Teething unduly protracted, early decay of teeth, curvature of the spine and limbs, enlargement of the joints and head, belly enlarged, appetite voracious, Diarrhoea.

Calc.-Phosph.—Very similar to the above, but Diarrhoea and prostration more marked.

Phosph.-Acid and *Phosph.*—With low fever, distended abdomen, Diarrhoea, milky urine, or turbid urine which deposits a white sediment.

Silicea—Skin morbidly susceptible to ulceration, scabby eruptions on the scalp, suppuration of glands, discharge from ears.

Sulphur—An excellent medicine to commence the treatment with, and to be employed for three or four days, when a remedy that has been productive of good has ceased to operate beneficially.

Accessory Means—Country air, dry, and bracing; abundance of sunlight, and out-of-door exercises. These wonderfully promote the cure, by imparting tone to the digestive organs, energy to the nervous system, and, in short, invigorating the whole constitution. Patients not able to walk should sit or recline in the open air, warmly clad, during portions of the day; this will aid recovery far more than passing the chief part of the day in the confined air of a sickroom. Exposure to ultra-violet rays acts in the same way as sunlight. Tepid or cold bathing, every morning, especially in salt water, followed by general massage for five or ten minutes, is valuable.

Diet—Nourishing food, well masticated, is of great importance. It should include milk, meat, eggs, animal fat (especially cod-liver oil and beef dripping), brown bread, etc. The administration of a moderate quantity of finely shaved juicy beef, once or twice a day, is advisable in some cases. *Malt* or *barely-food* is suitable for rickety children. If finely ground, the sediment from the husk need not be removed from the prepared food, as it is very nutritious, and rich in bone-forming materials. Boil four tablespoonfuls of *ground malt* in a pint of water for ten minutes. Pour off the liquid, and add an equal quantity of new milk. This food is very agreeable to children, and highly nutritious. An excellent food for rickety children is made by gently simmering groats in milk. A tablespoonful of groats is put into a vessel containing pint of milk; this is then placed in a saucepan or other vessel containing water, which is allowed to boil. When the milk has lost a quarter of its bulk, it should be strained, and is then ready to be given. The groats remaining behind are also an excellent food.

Surgical measures—If mechanical support be necessary for curvatures of the lower limbs, simple straight wooden splints, kept in place by a good bandage, are the best. But weakly children should be first treated by the administration of Cod-liver oil, and other remedies we have prescribed, and splints applied when the child's condition is improved, should they still appear necessary. As just stated, Cod-liver oil is an important remedy, but it should only be given in small doses, ten to twenty drops at first and the quantity gradually increased to a teaspoonful. Small pieces of ice put into each does render the oil almost tasteless. During its administration the evacuations should be examined, for the appearance and odour of the oil in them are signs that the quantity should be reduced.

TUBERCULOUS DISEASE OF BONES AND GLANDS

Definition—The old-fashioned terms *Struma* and *Scrofula*, interpreted in the light of modern knowledge, signify a constitutional disease, *Tuberculosis,* localizing itself especially in bones and glands. In children Tuberculosis shows itself seldom as Tuberculosis of the lungs ("Consumption" as it is popularly called), but very often as Tuberculosis of bones, glands, and membranes (especially the peritoneum—*Tuberculous Peritonitis,* and the covering of the brain—*Tuberculous Meningitis*).

Symptoms—There are two general types of the tuberculous patient: the one with coarse thick features, rough coarse dark skin, thick lips, sallow complexion; the other with fine delicate skin and features, blonde ("pink and white") complexion, long eyelashes, and downy growths of hair especially on the back. The local signs are swelling and pain in bones (as e.g. the limb bones of feet and hands, vertebrae) which, unchecked, go on to ulceration and discharge of tuberculous "pus"; swelling, usually at first painless, of glands, particularly in the neck, where they are readily seen and felt, but also (and quite as important) in parts where they can only be felt (e.g. the mesenteric and other glands in the abdomen—see page 80, *Consumption of the Bowels*), and in parts where they can be neither seen nor felt (e.g. the bronchial glands in the thorax). The glands in the neck and under the lower jaw are at first hard and the skin over them is not reddened. As they enlarge they tend to get softer and to reach the skin, reddening it. Unchecked they are then apt to "break down" and ulcerate the skin. Healing then leaves usually a ragged unsightly scar. To avoid this, when the skin is markedly reddened and pus or matter has evidently formed, the help of a surgeon should be sought. Much may be done by the use of homoeopathic remedies to prevent tuberculous glands reaching this state.

Cause—The tubercle baillus. This is partically always acquired—the "seed"; but there is very often a hereditary predisposition—the "soil." Predisposing conditions are the want of pure air, want of sunlight, and want of good food (especially of milk and animal fats) and any lowering illness, especially Measles and Whooping-cough.

Treatment—This disease is often very obstinate, and months, it not years, may elapse before a cure is effected. The most useful remedies are—*Ars.-Iod., Calc., Fer., Iod., Merc., Phosph.,* and *Sulph.* A dose need not be given oftener than night and morning.

Indication for the above and
other Remedies

Arsen.-Iod.—"It seems probable that in Arsenic Iodide we have a remedy most closely allied to manifestations of Tuberculosis" (*Boericke*). Profound prostration, rapid pulse, fever, loss of flesh, exhausting discharges from the bowels, night sweats.

Aurum—Various *affections of the bones*, and in case improperly dosed with *Mercury*. *Ferrum* and *China* are deserving of attention in like cases.

Belladonna—When sensitive organs are affected—such as the eye, the ear, and the throat; heat, redness, and *pain* in the eye, and *great intolerance of light*; neuralgic pains; sore throat, rendering swallowing difficult, painful swelling of the parotid and other glands, etc. (See "Mumps," page 64.)

Calcared Carbonica—General ill-health, enlarged abdomen, weakness of the bones, *slow dentition, strumous swellings,* great susceptibility to cold and damp, frequent discharge from the nose. When abundance of good food fails to induce a healthy state of the system—the child being pallid, cold, flabby, and dull—this remedy is of great service.

Ferr.-Iod.—Is of great value in the *anaemic,* impoverished, and cachectic conditions common in Tuberculosis, from imperfect assimilation of food.

Hepar Sulph.—Ulceration of the eyes; tendency to abscesses, great sensitiveness to cold.

Iod.—Enlargement of the glands, emaciated appearance, with hectic symptoms.

Iris.—*Scabby eruption* in lips, cheeks, ears, and head; frequent bilious Diarhoea.

Mercurius Biniod.—*Enlarged glands;* hard abdomen; various eruptions on the head, face, and ears.

Mercurius Sol. 6—Glandular inflammations with much

swelling and redness, the *pains* being *worse at night in bed,* particularly when the glands of the neck are swollen and painful, and there is inflammation of the eyes; *copious saliva;* disagreeable taste, and frequent and *unhealthy-looking foetid stools.*

Phos.—Frequently and easily disordered lungs; short, dry cough, tendency to Diarrhoea.

Silicea.—*Tuberculous ulcers* with callous edges; fistulous ulcers; *Otorrhoea;* tuberculous affections of the bone. It may follow *Calc.,* especially in diseases of the bones.

Sulphur—*Unhealthy skin;* Phlyctenular Conjunctivitis; humid eruptions behind, or purulent discharge from, the ears; swelling of the axillary glands, tonsils, nose, or upper lip; swelling of the knee, hip, or other joints; defective nutrition; colicky pains, mucous discharge, etc.

Fuller indications for many of the remedies will be found in the sections specially treating of the disorders mentioned in this section.

Accessory Means—In the treatment of strumous children three points are of prime importance—nourishing food, fresh air, and regular exercise. Proper attention to these are necessary, for medicines are not alone sufficient. The air of Margate and Ramsgate has the most wonderful effect on Scrofulous patients.

Food—The food should always be sufficient, nutritious and digestible, but not excessive. Beef, mutton and fowl are the best kinds of animal food; to these should be added plenty of eggs and milk, fat, bacon, and the ordinary articles of the mixed diet.

Cod-liver oil, as a supplementary article of diet, has a profound influence on tuberculous processes. It may be given in the absence of acute febrile symptoms, in small doses, three times a day. A teaspoonful is generally sufficient to begin with for a dose, and if it disagrees half a teaspoonful. Later the dose may be increased. Inunction with Cod-liver oil or with olive oil is also of great advantage.

Exercise—Moderate exercise in the open air is most essential. A bracing mountain or sea air, if it can be borne, is the best. A *cold* climate, if the child is warmly clothed, is generally favourable; but damp is injurious. The patient's room should also be uninterruptedly supplied with *pure air*. *Bathing*, both in fresh and salt water, is invaluable as a means of promoting a healthy action of the skin, and of imparting tone to the whole system. If sea-water cannot be obtained directly from the ocean, *Bumsted's* or *Tidman's sea salt* will form a valuable substitute.

Clothing should be adapted to the season, and be warm without being oppressive. The extremities especially should be kept warm. As a general rule flannel or wool should be worn. The linen should be frequently changed, always observing that it is put on perfectly *dry*.

Prevention—The prevention of tuberculous diseases consists not alone in the hygienic or medical treatment of the patients, but *primarily* in the correction of the habits and improving the health of the parents, more particularly in respect to the points referred to under "Causes."

TUBERCULAR MENINGITIS (Acute Hydrocephalus)

This disease is frequently fatal to tuberculous children, though all ages are liable to it. Its essentially morbid character consists in the growth of tubercle on the arachnoid membrane of the brain.

Symptoms—When occurring in children, the usual manifestations of the disease are—febrile disturbance, quick, irregular pulse; Vomiting; Constipation, the motions having the appearance of clay; red tongue; and continuous high temperature. The child manifests pain in the head, intolerance of light and noise; has disturbed sleep; grinds his teeth and is irritable: is unable to stand, from *vertigo*; and becomes generally feeble. He also desires to be quiet; has occasional delirium; looks old and distressed; suddenly cries out; and is very drowsy. Twitching and squinting may also occur. In unfavourable cases coldness of the extremities, clammy perspiration, an exceedingly rapid and feeble pulse, and death supervene.

Treatment—*Acon.*, followed by *Bell.*, and afterwards *Bry.* are the medicines in most repute in this disease.

Indications for the above and other Remedies

Acon.—Febrile disturbance, especially in the early stage.

Arsen.-Iod.—In the last state with marked prostration and emaciation.

Bell.—Red, hot face; heat of the head; bright or unusually dull eyes; intolerance of light and noise. *Calcarea Carb.* given in alternation with *Bell.* has restored desperate cases.

Bryonia—Suspicion of impending effusion on the brain.

Helleborus—Enlargement of the *fontanelles* (the open spaces in the heads of young children at the points of junction of the bones) from copious effusion, pulsation being discernible.

Hyoscyamus—Frequent starting, and picking with the finger.

Zincum—Paralysis of the brain; insensibility and involuntary evacuations.

Sulphur—During convalescence.

Iodoformum—"Should not be forgotten in the treatment of Tubercular Meningitis, both as a local application to the head and internally" (*Boericke*).

Accessory Treatment—This should include applications of cold water to the head, liquid diet, sponging the body with cold or tepid water followed by rapid drying, and *strict quietude*.

CONSUMPTION OF THE BOWELS

Definition—This is an old-fashioned term, and really covers several conditions, not all tuberculous, but conveniently considered together, viz (*a*) *Coeliac disease*, (*b*) *tuberculous disease of the mesenteric glands* (Tabes Mesenterica), (*c*) *tuberculous ulceration of the bowel*, (*d*) *tuberculous disease of the peritoneum* (Tuberculous Peritonitis). The last three of these, or any two of them, may co-exist.

Symptoms—First, Coeliac disease is a disease beginning in the second year, characterized by wasting, languor, abdominal distension, and a peculiar Diarrhoea of pale, offensive, very bulky, porridge-like stools. It is of very chronic course, liable to relapse, not fatal and not tuberculous though it often arouses a suspicion of Tuberculosis. It differs from *Tabes Mesenterica* in having no enlarged glands, and from Tuberculous Peritonitis in having no ascites (fluid in peritoneum).

Next Tabes Mesenterica is marked by anaemia and wasting, distension of the abdomen, enlargement of the deep glands of the abdomen (which may produce the effect of large tumours), a Diarrhoea of thin, offensive stools, and fever.

Thirdly, in tuberculous ulceration of the bowel there are similar characteristics, with more marked pain and tenderness, and tubercle bacilli in the stools.

Fourthly, in Tuberculous Peritonitis there are the same general features of fever, anaemia, emaciation, and abdominal distension and tenderness. There are also nausea, vomiting, and an alternation of constipation with Diarrhoea of pale, offensive motions. Two main types are distinguished, (a) the "wet," in which there is much *ascites*—the more favourable form, (b) the "dry" or *plastic* type, in which there is great thickening and adhesion of omentum and bowels, causing lumps and indurations as well as a general doughy feeling, together perhaps with enlarged glands.

Treatment—If seen early a few doses of *Sulphur,* followed by a course of *Calc.-Carb.*, or *Merc.-Bin.* will probably prove most beneficial.

Indications for the above and other Remedies

Aresenicum Iod.—Prostration, weakness, thirst, profuse Diarrhoea.

Calc.-Carb.—Well-marked scrofulous cachexia, swelling of glands, listlessness, aged expression.

Iodium—Diarrhoea, cough, night-sweats, and variable appetite.

Iodoformum—Chronic Diarrhoea, abdominal distention, enlarged mesenteric glands.

Merc.-Bin.—Profuse Diarrhoea, variable appetite, great distention and tenderness of abdomen, thirst.

Sulphur—In the first state and during convalescence.

Tuberculinum—In early stage, where the child (usually of fair complexion) is constantly catching cold. Early morning offensive Diarrhoea.

Accessory Treatment—The general treatment of the tuberculous forms of abdominal disease is much the same. The patient should receive an abundance of milk and fatty food, especially Cod-liver oil, also fruit; externally, fresh air and sunlight. A prolonged stay at the seaside, especially on the east coast of Kent, together with sea-bathing, is of the highest benefit. The patient should be warmly clothed, and in particular should not be allowed to conform to the prevalent practice of reducing the clothing of the lower limbs to a minimum. A flannel bandage should be worn round the abdomen. Massage, especially with Cod-liver oil, is good. In Tabes Mesenterica and Tuberculous Peritonitis it is good practice to rub in iodoform ointment. In Tuberculous Pertonitis with marked dropsy, operation (the letting out of fluid and letting in of daylight) often does a great deal of good. Such operation should be accompanied and followed by homoeopathic medication. The treatment of Coeliac disease differs from that of the other forms of abdominal disease in respect of diet. In Coeliac disease fat and starchy food must be severely restricted, and reliance largely placed on raw meat, raw meat juice, jellies, and malted foods (e.g. Mellin's biscuits, grape-nuts, Horlick's malted milk).

MUCO-PURULENT OPTHALMIA
(Phlyctenular Conjunctivitis)

Definition—Inflammation of the mucous membrane which lines the inner surface of the eyelids and the front part of the globe of the eye, occurring in delicate children, often of tuberculous stock, generally under eight years of age, and in your persons advancing towards puberty.

Symptoms—The prominent ones are—*dread of light; spasmodic contraction of the orbicularis palpebrarum muscle*, the lids being everted by the spasmodic action; *profuse flowing of tears*, which excoriate the cheeks; sensation as of grit in the eye. there are often such concomitants as styes, enlargement of the glands in the neck, sore ears, etc.

Cause—The *real* cause or "seed" is doubtless microbic, the "soil" often pre-tuberculous; the *exciting* causes are exposure to bright light, cold, and irritating vapours, neglect of cleanliness, etc.

Treatment—as a general rule it will be advisable to commence with *Sulphur*—a dose three times a day—and to continue it as long as it appears to be acting beneficially. But if no manifest improvement result in four or five days, *Mercurius Cor.* should be given at similar intervals.

Indications for the above and other Remedies

Arsenicum—Burning in the eyes; obstinate cases after the failure of other remedies.

Balladonna—As an intercurrent remedy if the eyelids be much swollen, and if an aggravation has resulted from exposure to cold.

Calcarea Carb.—When with the eye symptoms there are swollen glands in the neck and other marks of the scrofulous constitution.

Euphrasia—Profuse discharge of tears in addition to the other symptoms.

Mercurius Cor.—Extreme intolerance of light; small pustules at the junction of the cornea with the conjunctiva.

Sulphur—Chiefly useful when the inflammation of the eyes is the only sign of scrofulous taint.

Accessory Means—As a *lotion*, warm water should frequently be applied during the acute stage, or tepid milk-and-water previously boiled. Much comfort may also be derived from holding the eyes over the vapour from hot water. The eye should be protected by a shade from the sun and wind. Wholesome nourishing food, including Cod-liver oil, and pure country or sea air are essential.

Chapter III

DISEASES OF THE NERVOUS SYSTEM

CHRONIC HYDROCEPHALUS—"WATER ON THE BRAIN"

Definition—A collection of watery fluid within the ventricles of the brain. It occurs before the suture and fontanelles are closed, so that the bones yield to pressure from within. The disease may be congenital or acquired.

Symptoms—The most marked feature is the disproportion between the size of the skull and that of the face. The circumference of the head, which at birth is about fourteen inches, may reach thirty to forty inches. The face under it appears small and triangular. The sutures are widely separated, and the anterior fontanelle is very large and pulsating. The child is usually weak, emaciated, imbecile, and liable to develop Spastic Paralysis, Convulsions, and Epilepsy. From the chronic form blindness results very often.

Causes—Congenital Hydrocephalus is due to faulty development in pre-natal life. Acquired chronic Hydrocephalus is mostly due to posterior basic Meningitis, the endemic form of the epidemic Cerebrospinal Meningitis.

Treatment—In the early state *Bell.* will probably be the most useful medicine to give, followed by *Calc.-Carb.* or *Merc.-Sol.* 6, or alternated with it.

Indications for the above and other Remedies

Apis.—Urine scanty, throat oedematous, traceable to Scarlatina.

Arsen.-Iod.—Tubercular cachexia, with enlarged abdominal glands, cough, and inanition or prostration.

Belladonna—Convulsions, and other acute symptoms.

Calc.-Carb—Joints large, bones soft or curved, teeth delayed or decayed, nutrition defective, especially in strumous children.

Digitalis—Urine suppressed or scanty; circulation feeble; particularly suitable for children of drunkards.

Ferrum Iod.—A puffy, flabby state of the system, enlarged glands, hard abdomen, and pale, earthy complexion.

Helleborus—Head very large, or enlarging fast. Acute symptoms.

Mercurius Sol. 6.—Syphilitic cachexia.

Silicea—Tendency to suppuration, perspiration of the hand, and other symptoms like those under *Calc.-Carb.*

Sulph.—Tedious cases; skin day or covered with variuos eruptions.

Accessory Treatment—The most important points are—fresh air, out-of-door exercise, Cod-liver oil, and nourishing food.

INFANTILE CONVULSIONS—FITS

Definition—Violent, irregular contraction of the voluntary muscles, alternating with relaxation.

Symptoms—In simple cases there is slight twitching of the facial muscles, rolling of the eyes, and some difficulty or irregularity of breathing which soon pass off spontaneously. Severe cases are marked by sudden loss of consciousness, violent movements of the arms, legs, and head; turning of the eyes so that the white is visible, and the pupils almost invisible; pallor or redness of the face, lividity of the lips; clenching of the hands, the thumb being *under* the fingers; and bending of the great toes upon the soles of the *feet*. The fit may last for one or two minutes, when it passes off either altogether, or to recur after a longer or shorter interval. The slighter attacks are common to new-born infants.

Causes—The irritation of Dentition, or of Indigestion, Worms, etc.; a blow or fall; fright; disease of the brain, impure supply of blood to the brain, as in the eruptive fevers; feeble action of the heart; deficient supply of blood from defective nourishment; suppressed eruptions.

Treatment—If the exciting cause be known, the medicine most closely indicated in such a case should be administered, but if the cause cannot be ascertained. *Camphor* may be employed at once pending the arrival of professional assistance, or until the choice of the appropriate remedy can be made. The *Camphor* may be given by inhalation, or by putting a drop of the tincure on the tip of the little finger, and inserting it between the lips of the patient. After *Camphor*, *Bell.* and *Cham.* are the most important remedies.

Epitome of Treatment

From Teething—Acon., Bell., Cham., Kali Brom., Ver.-Vir.
From Mental Emotions—Acon., Opi., Coffea.
From Gastric Derangements—Nux V. (constipation), Ipecac. (vomiting), Puls. (from fatty food).

From Brain Disease—Acon., Bell., Gels., Hell., Hyos., Kali Brom., Ver.-Vir.

From Repelled Eruption—Ammon.-Carb., Bell., Bry.

From Worms—Calc.-C., Cina., Ign., Sulph.

Indications for some of the most useful Remedies

Aconitum—*Fever;* restlessness; fits caused by *fright* or excitement.

Belladonna—*Red Face;* brilliant eyes; heat of the head; starting at the least noise; rigidity of the whole body.

Bryonia—From repelled eruptions; cough and difficulty of breathing.

Camphor—*Depression of the fontanelles*—(For infants one or two drops on a little loaf sugar, which should be crushed and mixed, and s small quantity of the camphorated sugar placed on the child's tongue.)

Chamomilla—*Redness of one cheek,* the other being pale; twitching of the muscles of the face, sour vomiting.

Hyoscyamus—Much starting and twitching in sleep; heaviness of the head, and fretfulness.

Opium—Dark red or purple, swollen and hot face; turning the eyes upward; insensibility to light; *snoring breathing ;* suppressed urine; confined bowels.

Veratrum Viride—Convulsions following each other rapidly.

Accessory Treatment—The clothing should at once be loosened, the head raised, the face sprinkled with cold water, and fresh air be admitted. Should the child not at once recover, he should be placed in a *warm bath* at 90°, as follows—

The patient should be immersed in water up to the neck, and directly afterwards a towel or sponge, squeezed out of cold water, applied to the head; the cold towel or sponge may be applied for about two minutes, but the patient kept in the bath for five or ten minutes. The temperature should be *fully maintained*, by additions of hot water carefully poured down the side of the bath till the patient is taken out. The bath should be given in front of a good fire, and a warmed blanket be in readiness to wrap the child in directly he leaves the bath. The hot bath is of great service; it draws the blood from the over-loaded brain to the general surface of the body.

If there be sickness without vomiting, warm water should be administered, or the throat tickled with a feather. If the child's bowels are constipated, a simple enema should be given. When a nursing-mother becomes over-heated, or violently excited, her blood and milk and thereby poisoned. Under such circumstances the milk should be withdrawn, and the brain and blood allowed to cool down before nursing again, or serious or even fatal results may ensue. In some cases one or two doses of *Aconite* or *Opium* should be given to the mother.

Preventive—When there is a tendency to Convulsions, as shown by a foul tongue and breath, disordered evacuations, with screaming, restlessness, etc., the addition of *lime-water* to the child's milk (a tablespoonful to a feeding-bottle of milk) often acts as a preventive. It has been thought that the old remedy — *Hyd. cum creta*—owed its doubtful reputation to the quantity of chalk this preparation contained, the chalk neutralizing to a certain extent the acid secretions of the intestinal canal.

SPASMODIC CROUP—CHILD-CROWING
(Laryngismus Stridulus)

Definition—These names are applied to a disease quite distinct from the true Croup (see page 111), for it is a purely nervous affection, inducing *Spasm of the glottis*. It occurs in early childhood, before the end of the first dentition.

Causes—Child-crowing is essentially a nervous disorder, the one almost constant antecedent or concomitant of which is Rickets.

Symptoms—It comes on suddenly, most often in the night, with a spasm of the glottis. The child stops breathing, becomes livid and seems about to suffocate, when he gives a loud "crow." This inspiratory effort is followed by rapid recovery. The spasm may last a few seconds or it may last minutes. Death sometimes occurs in an attack.

Diagnosis from Croup *(Catarrhal Laryngitis)*—Laryngismus Stridulus is a nervous spasm that comes on suddenly, and is not usually or necessarily attended with hoarseness, cough, or fever.

Treatment—*Acon.* is of priceless value in Spasmodic Croup, and should be given before any other remedy—a dose every five or ten minutes, for three or four times, or until the spasm relaxes. *Bell.* is also of great service, and is preferred to *Acon.* by some physicians.

Indications for the above and other Remedies

Acon.—Is to be preferred if the skin be hot and dry, and the pulse hard, full, and accelerated.

Bell.—Much arterial and cerebral excitement.

Hep.-S.—To be used after *Acon.* or *Bell.* if wheezing or hoarseness is left after the spasm is relaxed.

Moschus—When the constriction in the larynx feels as if caused by the vapour of sulphur, and with inclination to cough.

Sambucus Nigra—Suffocating cough, waking the child up in the middle of the night, with wheezing and difficult breathing, but without Croup.

Spongia—An excellent remedy to be administered after *Acon.* or *Bell.*, and for some days—a dose three times a day.

Accessory Means—Fomentation to the throat, by means of a sponge wrung out of hot water; the warm bath; squeezing cold water on the child's face; making it retch by putting a finger or a feather down its throat; a whiff of chloroform; and the removal of any known existing cause, especially such as arise in the digestive organs.

EPILEPSY—FALLING-SICKNESS

Definition—Sudden and complete loss of consciousness and sensibility, with spasmodic contractions of the muscles, followed by exhaustion and deep sleep. The fit is often ushered in by a cry or scream, and the tongue is bitten unconsciously.

Premonitory Symptoms—An approaching seizure is sometimes announced by headache, shooting pains, giddiness, indistinctness of vision, sparks of various colours, strong odours, sneezing, strange tastes, hoarseness, humming noises, loud reports, irritability, dejection, and various illusions. But the most striking premonition is the *aura epileptica*, a peculiar sensation passing along the limbs, the head, or stomach, which, as soon as it stops, is followed by the fit.

Symptoms—The patient utters a loud, terrifying shriek, and falls convulsed and insensible. The movements of the head and neck and often most violent, one side being more affected than the other; the jaws are clenched, foam issues from the mouth, often tinged with blood from the tongue being bitten; the eyes are fixed and staring, or roll about; the hands are firmly clenched over the thumbs; urnien and faeces sometimes escape involuntarily; breathing is difficult, the face pale, the veins of the forehead distended; the heart's action violent and irregular, and death seems inevitable. After from one to three minutes the fit relaxes, leaving the patient insensible, and in a profound sleep. On awaking, the child generally seems bewildered.

There is a milder form, in which the child suddenly leaves of play, stands stupefied for a few seconds, the face turning pale, then resumes his play, as if nothing had occurred. This is *le petit mal* of the French, and may grow into the severer from, *le grand mal*, previously described.

Causes—Hereditary tendency: injury of the skull; local irritation, as a splinter or shot under the skin; tumours; inflammation; parasties in the brain; malformation of, or deposits in the skull; cutting teeth. The *exciting* causes in children are fright, fits of range, nervous perturbation, Hysteria, physical and psychical prostration. Fits are most likely to occur between the second and tenth years, during the period of the second dentition.

Other causes are—gastric disorder, the irritation of worms, repelled eruptions, especially about the head. This disease is more amenable to treatment in children than in adults; but hereditary tendency is always an unfabourable element in a case.

Treatment—1. *During the fit.*—It is very doubtful whether any medicine is of much service when given immediately before the occurrence of or during a paroxysm. 2. *Between the fits*—*Bell.*, *Calc.-Curb.*, and *Cuprum* have acquired the highest reputation in the treatment of this disease. A dose of the selected remedy may be administered once or twice a day.

Indications for the above and other Remedies

Acidum Hydrocyanicum—Recent Epilepsy.
Belladonna—Redness of the face, sparkling of the eyes, heat of the head, dilated pupils, complete loss of consci-

ousness, foam at the mouth, involuntary action of bowels and bladder.

Calcarrea Crab.—Especially useful when the fits depend upon the morbid influence of a scrofulous condition.

Chamomialla—Occurring in irritable children; the attacks often preceded by colicky pains, sour vomiting, and paleness of one cheek and redness of another.

Cina.—When the fits are evidently due to the irritation of worms.

Cuprum—Severe convulsions, the spasms usually commencing in the fingers or toes; salivation.

Ignatia—In attacks having an emotional origin and before the disease has become chronic.

Nux Vomica—Attacks preceded by Constipation and anger.

Stramonium—Recent Epilepsy caused by fright; Epilepsy in stammerers.

Sulphur—Arising from suppressed eruptions or discharges; also in scrofulous children.

Accessory Means—The patient's tongue should be put back into his mouth, and a cork or linen pad fixed between his molar teeth; he should be laid on a couch or rug, fresh air freely admitted around him, his head slightly raised, and all ligatures relaxed that interfere with circulation and breathing. Throwing cold water on the face does no good, and restraint should not be exercised beyond what is absolutely necessary. In Epilepsy preceded by the *aura,* a firm ligature applied above the part where the sensation is felt is said to prevent the attack. After the fit, the patient should be allowed to pass undisturbed the period of sleep which follows. Hygienic treatment, especially such as the causes of the disease suggest, is of great importance. Under this head we would prominently mention sponging the body, and especially the head, every morning with cold water, quickly followed by rapid and thorough drying. Shower-baths do not usually agree, and bathing in the open sea is obviously dangerous. All violent emotions, excesses of every kind and especially the precocious development or the unnatural excitement of the sexual instinct, must be strictly interdicted or prevented.

Regular out-of-doors exercise is beneficial, but it should never be carried too far, as fatigue often excites an attack. Epileptic patients require much *rest* and frequent change: boys and girls should not on any account sit at lessons for three or four consecutive hours. Studies and open-air recreations should be pleasantly blended.

Should fright, disappointment, anxiety, or other mental influences tend to keep up the disease, a thorough change is necessary, including change of residence, companions, and habits. "All ambitious intellectual exertion, especially rapid and discursive reading and writing against time, should be absolutely prohibited. But moderate employment of the thoughts, especially on familiar and interesting hobbies, is useful in preventing that stagnation or concentration of the mind upon itself which is so hurtful in all chronic complaints" (*Chambers*). Further, the mind requires pabulum, or food, and exercise for its healthy growth. The *diet* should be nourishing and taken regularly, in moderate quantities, including animal food once or twice a day. As the appetite is often voracious, it should be judiciously controlled. There is much to be said for a vegetarian diet.

INFANTILE PARALYSIS (Polio-myelitis)

Definition—A paralysis (not really "infantile," because affecting children above the age of one year) affecting one or more limbs, upper or lower; frequently only a group of muscles in one or more limbs.

Symptoms—The disease is ushered in with fever, perhaps sore throat, Convulsions, or gastric symptoms. On the subsidence of the fever it is found that the child cannot stand or walk, and has lost knee-jerk or knee-jerks, or has lost the power to move an arm. The affected parts are usually very tender at first. The initial paralysis is nearly always a good deal more extensive than what is found after, say, six or nine months. But recovery of muscular power is seldom complete. As all the muscles are not always paralysed to an equal extent, the limb may become contorted by the contration of those muscles which still retain power. Hence, in chronic cases, may result club-foot, drawing of the toes upon the sole of the foot, drawing up the leg, drawing together of the thighs, etc.

Cause—As the disease sometimes occurs in epidemic form, the cause must be microbic. There is reason to think that the germ gets access through the nasal or naso-pharyngeal mucous membrane, and therefore douching of these parts which an antiseptic lotion might be adopted as a preventive measure.

Treatment—In the early stage of the disease *Acon.* should be the medicine administered. In a day or two *Bell.* or *Gelsem.* will be more appropriate. Later on *Nux* or *Phos.* may be required. In all cases the limb must be kept warm with the greatest care; being placed frequently in a hot bath, and wrapped in wool. Afterwards *Lathyrus Sat.* may be given.

Indications for the above and other Remedies

Acontium—In recent cases, consequent upon cold, or attended with inflammatory disturbance.

Belladonna—Paralysis associated with Convulsions, flushed face, intolerance of light.

Gelseminum—When the symptoms combine those of *Acon.* and *Bell*.

Calcarea Carb.—Palsy, with general debility and malnutrition; enlarged glands, and other evidences or Scrofula.

Nux Vomica—Loss of power in the lower limbs, with coexisting Indigestion and Constipation.

Phos.—Following debilitating losses, such as Diarrhoea, etc.; resulting from fatty degeneration.

Rhus Tox.—The best remedy for the disease when occurring as a sequel of fever.

Accessory Means—Every effort must be made to raise the tone of the whole system by fresh air, out-of-door exercise, salt-water baths, etc. When there is much debility, *Cod-liver oil* is often of signal benefit. Massage and passive motion are also valuable accessories. In obstinate cases, *local galvanism* to the affected muscles will sometimes effect a cure. The daily application of faradization for weeks or even months may be necessary. If the disease has been neglected for several years, fatty degeneration may have taken place, in which case electricity is inadmissible.

CHOREA—ST. VITUS'S DANCE

Definitions—A disease characterized by involuntary convulsive muscular movements and ludicrous gesticulations, involving the face and limbs.

Symptoms—Twitching movements of the hands and arms, gradually extending to the muscles of the head, neck, and trunk. In some cases the patient can neither stand nor walk, and can with difficulty lie in bed. One side or both sides of the body may be affected. The movements generally cease during sleep; in severe cases they may be continued in sleep.

Causes—Rheumatism is the cause of Chorea in children. Chorea is, in fact, a rheumatic affection of the cortex of the brain. Exciting causes are mainly emotional, especially fright. But patients, of rheumatic constitution, seeing others suffering from the disease, are liable to voluntary or involuntary imitation.

Indications for Treatment

Aconitum—From fright or cold, especially if fever symptoms accompany the spasmodic movements.

Agaricus—In recent cases, especially if the child is very chilly and suffers from chilblains.

Cimicifuga—If associated with rheumatic pains, especially in head, back, and neck ("stiff neck").

Ignatia—From depressing emotions; in hysterical persons.

Additional Remedies—*Ars., Bell., Curprum, Hyos., Phos., Stram., Zincum, Tarantula, Mygale.*

Accessory Means—A *change of air* as well as of the general surroundings of the patient is frequently of great advantage. We have again and again found obstinate cases yield rapidly to this course when other courses had but partially succeeded.

Rest in bed for several days is often advisable; it secures a uniform temperature, and repose for the muscular and nervous symptoms: at the same time it reduces the wear-and-tear of the system to a minimum, and also isolates the child from other children.

The diet should be plain, sufficient, and taken regularly at three meals daily.

All excitement, including the excitement of school life, should be eliminated from the life of the chronic patient.

HEADACHE

Headache may be either a symptom of simple functional disturbance of the brain or other organs, or it may be an early symptom of disease of the brain.

Our chief object in this Section is to give directions for the cure of *simple* Headache, from whatever cause it may arise; and to point out the symptoms which indicate organic intercranial change. Diseases of the brain, especially organic, are most deceptive, and difficult of detection and diagnosis. They are prone to run a rapid course, and to end suddenly, and often unexpectedly, in death.

When a child complains of Headache, or if too young to complain, shows by his desire to lie down, or to have the head supported, by restlessness and peevishness, that his head aches, it is always well to inquire if he has had a fall upon, or any injury to, the head, been exposed to a hot sun or to great heat, or if he has taken indigestible food. Should the affection have no definable cause, and persist after the administration of the remedies prescribed, it is important that a physician should be at once consulted, as the headache may be due to Tuberculous Meningitis, Hydrocephalus, Syphilitic disease of the brain, etc.

Treatment—From headache arising—
From Exposure to Heat—Acon., Bell., Cactus, Glon.
From Indigestion—Iris, Nux, Plus.
From Injury—Arn.

Indications for the above Remedies

Aconitum—Throbbing pain, fever symptoms.
Arnica—Following an injury.
Belladonna—Pain in the temples, or the back of the head, red face, bright eyes, dilated pupils, starting and screaming in sleep.

Glonoine—Coming on suddenly; paleness of face; faintness and inability to hold the head erect.

Iris— With bilious Vomiting or purging.

Nux Vomica—With constipation; worse in the morning and in the open air; in girls and boys of a dark complexion.

Pulsatilla—Worse in the evening, relieved in the open air; in girls and boys of fair complexion.

Accessory Treatment—The *wet compress* in the form of a thick soft canvas cap, with an oiled-silk cover, is an admirable application in almost all kinds of Headache. When the head is very hot, cold affusions are highly advantageous, but the feet should be kept warm by friction, or by artificial heat. The patient should lie in a quiet room with a subdued light, and be protected from every kind of disturbance.

SLEEPLESSNESS

Sleeplessness is a symptom rather than disease *per se*. It may depend upon a disease—of which is forms a prominent symptom—or upon irritation of the nervous system, the excitement produced by strong emotions, or from the head being propped up too high. We purpose here to treat principally of the complaint as it occurs unconnected with any grave disease; but inasmuch as the remedies suitable for simple sleeplessness are often the most efficient in over-coming insomnia connected with serious disease, the latter will be incidentally mentioned.

Remedies—*Acontium*—Sleeplessness   from   fright, agitation, or anxiety, with *febrile heat.*

Belladonna—Great desire, but inability to sleep; fear, agitation, and frightful visions: continued crying without assignable cause; *heat and throbbing* in the head.

Coffea—Sleeplessness due to, or accompanied with,

agreeable excitement, laughter, playfulness, etc., and unaccompanied by feverishness. Over-active brain.

Hyoscyamus—Sleeplessness in sensitive or irritable children, from nervous excitement.

Ignatia—When due to *grief,* depressing emotions, or *Thread-worms.*

Nux Vomica—Flow of ideas preventing sleep; *Indigestion or Constipation.*

Opium—Hideous visions after a fright.

Pulsatilla—From repletion or *indigestible food.*

Accessory Means—When a child cannot fall asleep at the accustomed hour, he should be turned from the light, or the room should be darkened, quiet maintained, and the head a little lowered. Bathing the head and neck with cold water, and well drying by rubbing them with a rough towel, will often be useful. Smoothing back the hair with the hand, or singing in a low monotonous tone, has often a soothing effect. It is very important to ascertain if the child's feet are warm, and if necessary to make them so by warm applications or friction. If too many hours have elapsed since the child has taken food, a biscuit or two, with a little milk-and-water, may be all that is necessary to bring about the desired slumber. When the child starts in sleep and cries, refusing to be pacified, it is often best to wake him thoroughly from his half-sleeping condition, when the dreams and visions that disturbed him will probably not return.

Infants should early be accustomed to the habit of being *put to bed awake;* this proceeding will save the mother a great amount of trouble; at the same time, the habit involves the exercise of a certain amount of discipline that will aid in the formation of youthful character.

Chapter IV

Diseases of the Eye, Ear, etc.

PURULENT INFLAMMATION OF THE EYES OF NEW-BORN INFANTS (Ophthalmia Neonatorum)

This form of inflammation generally appears three or four days after birth; occasionally it may come on somewhat later.

The eyelids are the usual seat of the inflammation, but in some cases it extends to the eyeballs, when there is great danger of the sight being lost. The disease is the same as Purulent Ophthalmia in the adult, except as modified by the undeveloped tissues and rapid growth of the infant organism, and is usually more severe. It is the chief cause of blindness in the poor.

Symptoms—The eyelids become red and swollen, and are gummed together during sleep; light soon becomes painful, and the eyes are kept closed; after this a muco-purulent secretion is found, which gradually passes into a discharge of thick yellow pus, and when the eyes are cleansed they are seen to be so vascular as often to resemble crimson velvet; the cornea looks smaller than natural, and as if sunk in a pit. The infant is restless and feverish, and there is general wasting of the body. Unfortunately, the disease is often overlooked in its early state, or supposed to be due to a cold in the eye, which is expected to soon pass away; as a consequence, extensive and often irreparable mischief may result before treatment is commenced.

Diagnosis—The *purulent* character of the discharge distinguishes the disease from simple *Catarrhal Ophthalmia*.

Causes—The most frequent is contact during birth with leucorrhoeal or gonorrhoeal discharges in the vaginal passage. Other microbic causes; neglect of cleanliness; infection from another child suffering from the same disease. Irritation of the conjunctiva with soft or irritant soaps, spirits, etc., may be an accessory factor. It is most frequent in weakly infants, imperfectly nourished and breathing a bad air, and in infants prematurely born.

Treatment—A dose of *Argentum Nitricum* every two or three hours, as recommended by the late Dr. Dudgeon, is probably the best treatment that can be adopted. A lotion of the same remedy—one grain of the pure salt to three ounces of distilled water—may be used if necessary. Should no good result ensue, *Mercurius Corrosivus* may be given.

Indications for the above and other Remedies

Aconitum—If there be febrile disturbance.

Argentum Nit.—Well-marked and severe cases.

Belladonna—In slight attacks, with intolerance of light, and swollen eyelids.

Accessory Means—These consist essentially in the observation of *great cleanliness*, the eyes being gently sponged or syringed many times a day, and in slightly smearing the edges of the lids with olive-oil or cold-cream by means of a camel's-hair pencil. before the infant goes to sleep. It is important never to bathe the inflamed eyes with *cold* water, but always with tepid water, or tepid milk-and-water. Warm fomentations and sponging are highly beneficial. The child should be kept in an airy, warm, but not in a too brightly lighted room, till the inflammation is cured.

The *Preventive* measures must have for their object the improvement of the mother's health prior to parturition, including the arrest of the local symptoms which we have stated to be the most frequent cause of the disease. The eyes of all new-born infants should be carefully washed out with plain boiled water or weak boracic solution. Where the mother suffers from leucorrhoea or gonorrhoea, some 10 per cent. solution of *Argyrol* should be dropped into the infant's eyes immediately after birth.

CATARRHAL INFLAMMATION OF THE EYES
(Ophthalmia Simplex)

Ophthalmia is a general term for inflammation of the mucous membrane which lines the eyelids, and the front part of the eyeball.

Causes—The *real* cause is usually imcrobic. *Exciting* causes are colds, draughts, and damp; vicissitudes of temperature, easterly and north-easterly winds; strong light; heat, smoke, dust, or foreign bodies in the eye.

Symptoms—Itching or soreness in the ball of the eye; sensation as of sand under the lids; *redness of the eyes,* with swelling of the vessels; itching and pricking or shooting pains; pustules and scales on the lids; the pains increase in the evening, and on exposure to cold, and there is agglutination in the morning.

Treatment—In the early stages a few doses or *Acon.* followed by *Bell.* will often arrest the progress of the disease.

Indications for the above and other Remedies

Aconitum—White of eyes presents the appearance as if covered with a red network; fever.

Arnica—Inflammation from external injuries.

Belladonna—Pain, redness, and swelling; throbbing in the temples; flushed cheeks, glistening eyes, and intolerance of light. Often used after *Acon.*

Hepar Sulphur—After the acute symptoms have yielded to the remedies prescribed above; Chronic Ophthalmia, with agglutination of the lids at night.

Mercurius Cor.—*Copious discharge* from the eyes with much *pain.*

Sulphur—*Frequent relapse in scrofulous children.* It may follow other remedies after the more urgent symptoms have subsided.

Additional Remedies—*Ars.* (for old standing cases); *Arg.-Nit.* (with purulent discharge); *Calc.-Carb.* (in scrofulous patients); *Phos.* (obstinate cases in consumptive patients).

Accessory Measures—If inflammation has been caused by sand, dust, lime, flies, or hairs of the lids, the irritating body should be immediately removed; and if the inflammation be considerable, a shade should be worn. To prevent the eyelids from being cemented together in the morning, they should be smeared with a little olive-oil or create, by means of a camel's-hair brush at bedtime, or a wet compress may be worn over the eyes at night. The eyes should be bathed with tepid water; and strong light and exposure to cold avoided till the inflammation subside. Children predisposed to Ophthalmia should be guarded against easterly and north-easterly winds. In mild but persistent cases of the disease, in which the ordinary remedies are availing, some constitutional derangement may be suspected, and must be removed before the ophthalmic symptoms will yield.

STYE

Definition—A small absces which forms round an eyelash, due to microbic infection.

Symptoms—Itching, heat, pain, sometimes slight fever, Styes are apt to be multiple and to keep recurring.

Cause—Microbic. Often associated with general debility and poor health; also with microbic infection elsewhere, such as boils and acne.

Treatment—*Acon.*, followed by *Puls.*, will often remove the stye if given sufficiently early. After this *Staphysagria* may be given.

Indication for the above and other Remedies

Aconitum—Pain, fever, restlessness.

Hepar S.—When suppuration has begun. Especially *upper* eyelid.

Pulsatilla—Especially *lower* eyelid.

Sulphur—During convalescence, and as preventive.

Accessories—Bathe the eyelid with very hot water several times a day, or apply a hot compress. If the stye does not readily burst, prick with a sterilized needle and let the matter out.

EARACHE (Otalgia)

Acute pain in the ear is not uncommon in children. This may be due to an inflammatory condition (e.g. a boil), or a foreign body, in the external meatus. More often it is due to an inflammation extending from the naso-pharynx along the Eustachian tube to the middle ear (*Otitis Media*); hence the common association with colds in the head and adenoids. It also occurs as a complication of other diseases, as Measles, Scarlet fever, Diphtheria, Influenza, Pneumonia, Whooping-cough, etc. In acute Tonsillitis there is often a sharp pain shooting into one or both ears, especially on swallowing.

Symptoms—The ordinary earache due to catarrhal inflammation of the Eustachian tube and middle car consists of a severe aching, throbbing pain, accompanied by some tenderness and sense of fullness in the ear, and usually by more or less deafness. The deafness and stuffed-up feeling in the ear is generally relieved temporarily by blowing down the nose with the nostrils closed, when a cracking is heard in the ear. In severer forms the pain may radiate upwards or forwards, or backwards and downwards into the neck, and there is tenderness over the mastoid process. The temperature may rise to 103°. The symptoms are all aggravated at night. If taken in time and properly treated, the otitis should not go on to suppuration. When suppuration takes place, the membrane tympani ("drum") is not only red but bulges outwards. Paracentesis or puncturing of the membrane should then be done under an anaesthetic. If left to itself, it will burst on the third or fourth day.

Diagnosis—In *infants* suffering from Otitis Media there may be Vomiting, Convulsions, and head-retraction, and the case may easily be diagnosed as acute Meningitis if the ear is not examined. Otitis Media is one of the complications of Pneumonia, and may then be present without pain or symptoms pointing to the ear. It may also at times exist independently, with no symptom but fever. In case of obscure fever the ears should always be examined.

Indications for Treatment—*Aconitum* —Pain, soreness, and throbbing in the ear; sensitiveness to noise; red, shining swelling of the meatus; feverishness.

Belladonna—When the head is much involved and the patient delirious—to be given either alone or alternately with *Acon.* or *Merc.-Sol.*

Chamomilla—Earache of nervous, irritable children, with one cheek red and hot.

Mercurius Cor.—After suppuration has taken place.

Merc.-Sol.—Catarrhal earache without suppuration.

Pulsatilla—In less acute and more persistent forms of the disease.

Sulphur—Chronic or recurring inflammation, especially in scrofulous patients.

Accessory Treatment—Plantago ø, diluted with an equal quantity of hot water and dropped into the ear. Warm olive oil dropped into the ear. The heart of an onion made very hot, or a tiny muslin bag containing hot salt, may be inserted into the external meatus, with great relief of pain, and a bran poultice may be put over the whole ear.

An inflammatory condition of the external meatus should be treated similarly, and *Belladonna*, *Hepar S.*, or *Merc.-Sol.* given internally. If the trouble is due to foreign bodies (e.g. peas, pips, insects), these must be removed by syringing.

DISCHARGE FROM THE EAR (Otorrhoea)

Definition—Wax (cerumen), more liquid than usual, may flow from the ear; blood too, as a result of fracture of the base of the skull or of rupture of the drum (*Membrana tympani*), may flow from the ear. But the term Otorrhoea is generally applied to a discharge of pus, muco-pus, or sanguineo-pus, nearly always offensive, chronic in its nature, and resulting from suppurative Otitis Media—often a sequel of Scarlet fever or Measles, and not rarely of tuberculous disease.

Indications for Treatment

Arsenicum—Old standing cases in delicate children; excoriating discharges.

Calc.-Carb.—Tedious cases in tuberculous children.

Hepar S.—Discharge of pus and blood; and when the patient has been dosed with Mercury.

Mercurius Cor.—Thick, bloody, foetid discharge, tearing pains in ear and side of head, swelling and tenderness of glands about the ear.

Mur.-Ac.—Following Scarlet fever.

Pulsatilla—Especially after measles or Mumps.

Sulphur—In cases similar to those calling for Calc.-Carb.

Additional Remedies—*Aurum, Iod. Kali Hyd., Merc.-Iod. Nit.-Ac.*, and *Sil*.

Accessories—The intractable character of this affection is often in great measure due to the neglect of that strict cleanliness which is indispensably necessary. A little fine wool, frequently changed, should be put into the ear, which should be gently syringed out with hydrogen peroxide (mixed with ten or twelve parts of water) three or four times a day.

The improvement of the general health of the patient is a point of great importance. To this end, change of air is often necessary; *country air*, in a dry, salubrious district, or, in the autumnal months, *sea air*, is generally of marked utility. *Cod-liver oil* is also strongly recommended.

GENERAL MANAGEMENT OF THE EAR

Sudden Violent Noises—It is very important to avoid the exposure of children to acute and extreme sounds, especially to those of firearms, which may occasion serious disorders, either rupturing the drum of the ear, or giving an injurious shock to the brain. When children have to be exposed to violent sounds, a little cotton-wool should be introduced into each ear to guard the drum of the ear from the painful impression of a too acute shock. This precaution is increasingly important in illness, especially in diseases which involve the nervous system.

Wet or Damp Ears—Imperfectly drying the head and ears of children after washing is sometimes a cause of Otitis Media and Deafness. It is the more necessary to guard against this danger if there already exist any discharge from, or other disorder of, the ear. The strictest care should be taken to dry the hair and ears *thoroughly* after bathing.

Twisted corner of towel not to be used—The introduction of the screwed-up corner of a towel, and twisting it round in the ear, does much harm. It forces down the wax upon the membrane, irritates the passage, and causes small flakes of skin, which dry up and become hard, so that pain, inflammation, and deafness may ensue. Washing should only extend to the external surface as far as the finger can reach, and the screwed-up corner of a towel should never be used for cleaning the cavity of the ear.

Boxing the Ears—Parents, governesses, and others who have the care of children, should be aware of an accident likely to result from blows on the head or boxing the ears, namely, rupture of the *membrana tympani*, a membrane which closes the bottom of the meatus, and is stretched something like the parchment of a drum. Sometimes incurable Deafness or hardness of hearing is the result. Rupture of this membrane may be recognized by a sense of shock in the ear, Deafness, and a slight discharge of blood from the orifice; and if examined by an ear speculum, the rent may be seen. For this injury a weak *Arnica lotion* should be employed, and the little patient should enjoy absolute *rest* for two or three days.

Foreign Bodies in the ear—The introduction of foreign bodies into the ear is no rare occurrence in children. Such substances, although they do not always give rise to mischief, should be removed at once by syringing with warm water. When insects find their way into the ear, they may be similarly dislodged.

Deafness not Stupidity—Another point of considerable importance is that a child should not be thought to be stupid or obstinate simply because he is deaf.

EPISTAXIS—BLEEDING FROM THE NOSE

This is generally a trifling ailment in children enjoying fair health, and requires no treatment, ceasing spontaneously in a few minutes.

When, however, it occurs in delicate children, when if recurs frequently, or when due to injury, treatment may be necessary.

Symptom—Giddiness, weight or oppression in the forehead, may precede the bleeding. In some cases the blood passes backward into the stomach, when it may, without careful investigation, be mistaken for haemorrhage from the lungs or stomach.

Causes—Injuries; *congestion* of the head from coughing, passion, etc.; thinness of the blood; weakness of the lining membrane of the nose, etc.

Indications for Treatment

Aconitum—Epistaxis from excitement or passion.

Arnica—From a blow or other injury.

Belladonna—When preceded by a throbbing headache. redness of the face, and brightness of the eyes.

China—When weakness results from loss of blood.

Hamamelis—Blood oozing slowly, drop-by-drop; not bright red.

Millefolium—Red blood flowing without apparent casuse.

Phosphorus—Bleeding from the nose when there are bruise-like marks (ecehymosis) on the body.

Accessories—The application of cold water, ice, or a cold iron to the forehead, neck, or back; holding the arms above the head for a few minutes, or pressing with the extended fingers horizontally across the cheekbone, just above the bleeding nostril. These means will rarely prove insufficient; but should they do so, a piece of lint may be rolled into the shape of the nostril, saturated with *Hamamelis* and twisted rather tightly into the bleeding nostril or nostrils, first removing any clots of blood there may be present.

This treatment is recommended not only on account of the styptic qualities of the remedy, but also for the mechanical support of the tightly-fitting plug. The child should be placed in a recumbent posture, in a cool room.

Chapter V

DISEASES OF THE RESPIRATORY SYSTEM

CROUP (Catarrhal or Inflammatory Croup)

Definition Inflammation of the mucous lining of the larynx and traches, with swelling from effusion into their sub-mucous areolar tissue, and secretion of tenacious mucus.

The essential nature of Croup is a catarrhal inflammation affecting the above organs, without the formation of any false membrane; when the membranous exudation does take place the disease is Diphtheria.

Causes—1. *Predisposing*—The comparative smallness of the larynx and trachea in infancy and early childhood. After the third year the calibre of the trachea enlarges rapidly, and the liability to Croup correspondingly diminishes. There is also a clear predisposition to it in some patients and families. The existence of "tonsils and adenoids." 2. *Exciting*—Exposure to cold, sudden changes of temperature, wet feet, poor and scanty food, especially the adoption of improper diet on weaning, keeping a child in a room the floor of which has been newly washed, dark, damp, low-lying localities. The disease is most frequent in winter and spring.

Symptoms—The *early* symptoms resemble those which initiate and attack of Measles—fever, hoarseness, and a *dry barking cough* of that distinctive character which necessarily occurs when the *rima glottidis* (opening between the vocal cords) is contracted. Indeed, this cough is the characteristic symptom, and probably exists two or three days before it is sufficiently marked to excite maternal alarm. But to educated ears the cough is characteristic almost from the commencement; and if the child be requested to take a deep breath the harsh sound completes the diagnosis.

The accession of the *alarming* symptoms generally occurs suddenly, and often in the night, the mother dating the attack from the commencement of the danger. The symptoms are very severe, but aggravated in frequent paroxysms; there is great difficulty of breathing from the congestion and swelling of the lining membrane of the larynx, and the diminution of the chink at its outlet, so that the child throws its head back to put the parts on the stretch; respiration is "crowing," and every breath becomes increasingly difficult, and the turgescence of the face and neck shows that an insufficient supply of air enters the lungs notwithstanding the severity of the respiratory efforts; the cough is loud and brazen, the voice is hoarse, or absent, the pulse quick, and the skin hot and dry.

In fatal cases, the lips and face become increasingly purple, the pulse smalll and thready, the lungs congested, and the patient dies from suffocation. In some cases death is preceded by Convulsions.

Diagnosis—The conditions from which "Croup" (Catarrhal or Acute Laryngitis) may need to be distinguished are *Diphteria, Laryngismus Stridulus,* and *Congenital Laryngeal*

Stridor. It is distinguished from *Diphtheria* (sometimes with great difficulty, the signs of obstruction being the same, whether the obstructing agent be merely inflammatory swelling of the mucous membrane or an actual membrane) by the facts that (*a*) a disease setting in acutely, abruptly, and dramatically is more likely to be Croup; setting in insidiously, Diphtheria, (*b*) while the temperature may well be higher in Croup, the constitutional disturbance is greater in Diphteria, (*c*) there is less cough and more loss of voice in Diphteria than in Croup—"Diphtheria is the more *silent* disease" (Hutchison). Croup is distinguished from *Laryngismus Stridulus* (see page 88) by the facts that in the latter there is no preliminary fever, catarrh or illness, the whole attack is over in a few seconds, and there is a history or evidence of Rickets. *Congenital Laryngeal Stridor,* in which the infant always makes a curious crowing or purring sound in breathing, is readily distinguished from Croup by the facts that the "crowing" is practically continuous, that the condition is congenital, and that it disappears spontaneously by the end of the first year.

Danger—This aries from the narrowing of the aperture for breathing consequent on the congestion and effusion present. The same amount of effusion into the submucous areolar tissue elsewhere would be of no grave consequence. This danger is diminished just in proportion as the cough becomes looser, and the secretion of the air-passages becomes thinner and more easily removed.

Treatment—As in all other inflammatory diseases, *Aconite* is here the leading remedy. It should be given every fifteen or twenty minutes for three or four times, and then every half-hour, until some marked impression is made upon the fever symptoms. *Spongia* may then be submitted for it, or the two medicines may be given alternately at intervals of an hour or two, as long as may be necessary.

Indications for the above and
other Remedies

Aconitum—Always in the early stage, and when there are any febrile symptoms, with short, dry cough, and hurried and laborious breathing.

Ant.-Tart.—When there is much oppression on the chest, copious *phlegm*, impeded respiration, and inclination to vomit.

Hepar S.—After the subsidence of the fever, when there is loose metallic cough, with rattling in the chest, and difficult expectoration.

Iodium—For scrofulous children especially. Hoarse, hollow, ringing, whistling cough, with pain in chest, and laboured breathing.

Spongia—For symptoms resembling those of *Iod.*

Sulphur—During convalescence.

Accessory Measures—During the treatment, everything likely to excite or irritate the patient should be avoided. He may have a partial or compete warm bath; his throat should be fomented by means of sponges or cloths squeezed out of *hot* water, and a compress or flannel applied to the part when not fomenting; the feet and general surface of the body kept warm, and the air of the apartment raised to about 65° Fahr., and this temperature uniformly maintained by day and night. The air should also be *moist* as well as warm. Steam may be inhaled, either alone or mixed with the remedy that is being administered. A few drops of the strong tincture of the remedy required may be dropped into a small tin kettle, kept boiling over the fire or over the flame of a spiritlamp, and fixing a tin or paper tube to the spout, convey the vapour close for the patient to inhale. In very bad cases a sort of tent should be formed over the patient's bed, and the steam conducted under it by a tube.

COLD IN THE HEAD, SNIFFLES (Coryza)

An inflammatory affection of the mucous lining of the nose, attended with abnormal secretion, which is occasionally so profuse as to interfere with breathing and suckling. In infants the disease is usually termed *sniffles*.

Causes—Exposure to draughts and cold, sudden changes of temperature, wet feet, inherited Syphilis (in infants).

Symptoms—Cold in the head usually comes on with slight shiverings, pain or a feeling of weight in the head, redness or itching of the eyes, obstruction of one or both nostrils, with an increase of the natural secretion of the parts, the discharge being a thin acrid fluid. If now neglected, these symptoms may be soon followed by sore throat, mucous discharge, hoarseness, sneezing, dry cough, chilliness, general weakness, more or less fever, quick pulse, and loss of appetite.

Treatment—In the very early stage *Camphor* should be administered. To infants it may be given by inhalation. A drop or two of the tincture should be put into a teaspoon and held near to the nostrils for a minute or longer, and repeated every twenty minutes for three or four times. To older children it may be given on sugar. Should this medicine fail to check the progress of the disease, some other will have to be had recourse to.

Indications for the above and other Remedies

Aconitum—In the early stage, especially if there be any febrile symptoms, swelling and redness of the lining membrane of the nostrils.

Arsenicum—Watery, excoriating discharge.

Camphor—Only useful in the chilly state.

Dulcamara—When brought on by damp.

Euphrasia—With copious watery discharge from the eyes.

Mercurius Sol. 6—In the profuse "running cold," as also in cases which the discharge is semi-purulent, this medicine is most efficacious.

Nux Vomica is the established remedy for the "stuffy cold."

Accessory Treatment—The child should remain in a room the atmosphere of which is of a comfortable, uniform temperature. A warm bath should be given on going to bed, and the child well wrapped in an extra blanket, so as to favour the free action of the skin; this is still further promoted by drinking freely of cold water during and after the bath. In the case of infants their noses should be frequently smeared with simple cerate, cold-cream, or tallow, to prevent the discharge from forming into hard crusts. In chronic obstinate cases the interior of the nostrils may be syringed with a weak solution of *Carbolic Acid*. It suckling be difficult or impossible, the milk should be drawn, and the infant fed with it by means of a spoon till the complaint be modified.

Prevention—Except before the third month, and for decidedly delicate children, rapid *cold bathing* of the whole body is a grand method of preventing children from being chilled by exposure to cold air, which is otherwise beneficial. For delicate children, tepid may be used at first, and gradually reduced to cold, and the bathing done very *quickly*. They should also be exposed to the *open air daily*, which tends to strengthen the body to resist atmospheric changes. Children should be *properly clothed*, especially the lower limbs and abdomen. Lastly, infants should be taught to use the *nostrils for breathing in sleep* instead of the mouth. This cannot be done too early, for the habit is difficult of acquirement if neglected till adult life.

ACUTE BRONCHITIS

Definition—Acute inflammation of the mucous lining of the bronchi—the air-tubes of the lungs. It is a *diffused disease*, involving more or less the smaller tubes of both lungs, thus differing from cold or catarrh, which only affects the lining memberane of the nose, throat, and eyes. When the upper portion of the chest is chiefly affected, patients often describe it as a *"Cold in the chest."*

Bronchitis is one of the most important diseases of early childhood, on account of its frequency, its liability to complication with Pneumonia, and the danger from suffocation which the accumulated mucus involves.

Causes—Exposures to cold draughts of air, to keen and cutting winds, or sudden changes of temperature; insufficient clothing; inhalations of dust, smoke, or other irritative substances. Bronchitis also arises during the course of other diseases—Measles, Whooping-cough, etc.—especially in weakened children. It is a common complication of Rickets.

Symptoms—Bronchitis usually begins with the symptoms of a common cold—feverishness, Headache, lassitude, cough, etc. These are soon attended with a feeling of tightness or constriction in the chest, especially the front portion; the breathing becomes oppressed and huried, with wheezing or whistling sounds; there is severe cough, which is at first dry, but is afterwards attended with viscid and forthy expectoration, subsequently becoming thick, yellowish, and purulent. The pulse is frequent, often weak; the urine scanty and high-coloured; the tongue foul; there are throbbing pains in the forehead, and aching pains n the eyes, aggravated by the cough, with other symptoms of fever. Nursing children suck with difficulty, or do so eagerly for a short time, and then desist from interrupted breathing, throw the head back, and commence coughing or crying.

The unfavourable symptoms are—*cold* perspirations covering the skin; pale and lived cheeks and lips; cold extremities; rapid respirations; the nostrils being widely dilated at each breath; drowsiness; *extreme prostration;* rattling, and a sense of suffocation in the throat; and complete insensibility, ending in death. Convulsions towards the end of an attack generally indicate collapse of the lung, and impending death. In favourable cases, the disease begins to decline between the fourth and eighth day, and under good treatment soon disappears.

Treatment—At the commencement of the disease *Aconitum* given at once, and repeated every hour or two hours, may arrest the attack in a very short time; but should it fail to do so, or the disease have advanced considerably before attention has been called to it, either *Ant.-Tart.* or *Kali Bichrom.* will have to be administered alone, or, if there be fever symptoms, alternately with *Aconitum*, at intervals of two hours or so.

Indications for the above and other Remedies

Aconitum—A short, hard cough, tickling of the pit of the windpipe and chest, burning and soreness of the chest on coughing, frontal headache, febrile symptoms.

Antimonium Tart.—*Weezing in chest;* paroxysms of *suffocative* cough, with copious loose expectoration, sickness bring often induced by the accumulation of mucus: dyspnoea, palpitation, and headache.

Bryonia—Especially valuable when rheumatic pains in the muscles were present before, or are present during, the attack.

Kali Bich.—When the expectoration is very stringy and tenacious.

Phos.—May be required if the inflammation extends to the substance of the lungs.

Accessory Measures—The patient should be kept in a warm atmosphere (65° to 70°), in a tent, with a bronchitis kettle, and encouraged to drink freely of hot liquids, especially hot lemonade. Ventilation of the room should not be neglected. Hot linseed-meal poultices applied to the back, *not to the chest*, are beneficial.

Diet—During an attack, gum-water, barely-gruel, beef-tea, jelly, etc. In feeble children, exhaustion is liable to come on, requiring nutritious support. During convalenscence, undue exposures must be guarded against until the constitution has been strengthened and inured by warm bathing, gradually reduced to cold as the reactive power of the child permits.

INFLAMMATION OF THE LUNGS (Pneumonia)

Definition—An acute inflammation of the lung tissue, accompanied by high temperature and very rapid respiration.

Varieties—Pneumonia is either *primary* (in which case it is generally *lobar*, i.e. it involves the whole of a lobe or more than one lobe) or *secondary* ("consecutive" to Measles, Diphtheria, Whooping-cough, ect.—in which case it is generally lobular and occurs in patches in the lung, developing upon a bronchitis and hence commonly called *Broncho-Pneumonia).* Lobar Pneumonia is most frequent in children between one and two, and it is a far less serious complaint than Broncho-Pneumonia, which often attacks infants.

Symptoms—The onset of *Lobar Pneumonia* is usually abrupt, with shivering and a sharp rise of temperature. Often there is vomiting to begin with, or even Convulsions. "A

deceptive onset of Pneumonia is with drowsiness"
(Hutchison). Respiration is rapid out of proportion to the
rapidity of the pulse, and expiration is apt to be grunting and
accompanied by an expansion of the *aloc nasi*. There is
frequent short, dry, painful cough and very sticky rust-
coloured sputum, which, however, children under three
seldom expectorate. There are often "water-blisters" on the
lips (*Herpes Labialis*). Physical signs are often in children very
indefinite at the onset of the disease, and diagnosis has to be
made upon the strength of the general evidence. In
favourable cases, resolution takes place by *crisis* on any day
from the fifth to the ninth, the temperature coming down
with a steep drop, together with pulse and respiration. Lobar
Pneumonia is not nearly so serious in children as it is in
adults—delirium and cardiac failure, for instance, are seldom
seen in children.

The onset of *Broncho-Pneumonia* is apt to be insidious. It is
usually secondary to a Bronchitis following on, or complicating, some such disease as Measles or Whooping-cough,
and it is often very difficult to be sure when the Bronchitis has
become a Pneumonia. Sustained high temperature, very rapid
respiration and cyanosis indicate Pneumonia. The
temperature is more apt to oscillate widely in Broncho-
Pneumonia than in Lobar Pneumonia, and it ends by lysis,
that is, by a gradual decline spread over two or three days.
The chief difference between the two forms of Pneumonia is
that Broncho-Pneumonia is vastly the more serious and fatal
disease.

Causation—The real cause of Lobar Pneumonia is the
pneumococcus; of Broncho-Pneumonia, occasionally the
pneumococcus, but more often a sterptococcus. The main
exciting cause, apart from an antecedent disease, is chill.

Treatment—If administered early, and every two hours,
Acon. will often be quite sufficient to check the advance of

the disease. If it fail to accomplish this, *Phosph.* should be given, either alone or in alternation with *Acon.*, at intervals of about two hours. Rarely any other medicines will be required.

Indications for the above and other Remedies

Aconitum—Fever symptoms, short rapid breathing, full pulse; in the early stage, and alternately with other medicines.

Ant.-Tart.—When the disease follows a cold in the head or Influenza, this medicine is usually found most beneficial. The expectoration is copious and free.

Belladonna—Short, dry cough, flushed face, headache. Seldom called for.

Bryonia—When the inflammation extends to the pleura, and there is consequently sharp stitching pain in the side, making movement and respiration painful. Goes very well in alternation with *Aconite* at the outset.

Phosphorus—Rusty-coloured sputa, difficult breathing, pain under the breast bone.

Sulphur—During convalescence.

Accessory Means—The child should be placed in a well-ventilated *warm room* (60° to 65°), and have only light bed-coverings; for cold air irritates the lungs, and heavy bed-clothes render the skin hotter and drier, and add to the discomfort and danger of the patient's condition. A light pneumonia-jacket of Gamgee tissue may be fitted to the patient. Heavy poultices are to be avoided—at any rate for the chest. Antiphlogistine is better than poultices, and for relief of pain is excellent. The patient should be kept very quiet and have milk-and-water, pain water or lemonade, etc.

INFLAMMATION OF THE PLEURA (Pleurisy)

Definition—Acute inflammation of the covering of the lungs and lining of the chest, usually affecting one side only. When uninflammed, the above membrane has a smooth, lubricated surface to facilitate the free movement of the lungs; inflammation destroyes this polished surface, so that any movement of the lungs, as in breathing or coughing, becomes difficult and painful.

Symptoms—Pleurisy generally comes on quickly and violently, with chills, and severe *stabbing pains* in the chest. The character of the cough, breathing, and pain reveals very much as to the variety of the inflammation of the chest from which the child is suffering. In Pleurisy the breathing is *hurried*, the child does not take a full, deep breath, and breathing is frequently *interrupted* by a *stitch* or *catch*, or by *cough*, which is frequently short and dry, and occassions a *sharp stabbing* pain below the nipple, about the fifth or sixth rib. Pain referred to the epigrastrium with marked oppression of breathing points to diaphragmatic Pleurisy, that is, inflammation of the pleura overlying the diaphragm. There is a parched tongue; flushed face; hard, wiry, quick pulse (about 100 in the minute); scanty, high-coloured urine; and the patient desires to lie on the affected side, or on the back.

The inflammation terminates in one of the following ways: by *resolution*, when the two surfaces of the pleura regain their natural smooth character, or the inflamed and roughened surfaces becomes more or less *adherent*; or *effusion* takes place, and a dropsical fluid separates the surface—a condition known as pleural effusion. Where there is much fluid effused there is great difficulty of breathing, and the lung becomes collapsed.

A professional examination of the chest is necessary to arrive at a correct disgnosis, otherwise it is often impossible to distinguish between *real* and *false Pleurisy*, or between this and other chest inflammations. False Pleurisy or Pleurodynia ("pain in the side") may mimic Pleurisy remarkably, but it is generally without fever, and on ausculation of the chest the friction sounds of Pleurisy are not heard. *Bryonia* and *Cimicifuga* are the remedies for this condition.

Causes—Exposure to atmospheric changes, and checked perspiration, especially in persons of feeble constitution. Pleurisy is also liable to arise during the course of fevers, or from the extension of inflammation from a neighbouring organ to the pleura; or it may be set up by mechanical injuries. It is important to remember that a large number of so-called simple pleurises are really tuberculous.

Treatment—If administrated early *Acon.* may alone be sufficient. If it does not quickly relieve, *Bryonia* will have to be substituted. A dose of the selected medicine should be given every hour or two hours, according to the urgency of the case.

Indications for the above and other Remedies

Acontium—Much fever, dry cough, in the early stage before adhension or effusion.

Bryonia—Short, laboured, anxious, *catching breathing*, preformed almost entirely by the abdominal muscles; frequent *cough*, which *shakes* and *pains* the side, either dry or with expectoration of glairy mucus; weariness, irritability, and restlessness.

As long as the febrile symptoms continue, *Acon.* may be alternated with *Bry.* These remedies often suffice to cure the disease in a day or two; or, if given early and at short intervals, in a few hours.

Sulphur—During convalescence, and to *prevent relapse*.

Accessory Means—Practically the same as for Pneumonia (see page 119). When effusion has occurred, and there is no evidence of absorption taking place, the Pneumatic *Aspirator** should be employed to evacuate the pleural contents without delay, especially when there is much dyspnoea, and when the collection of fluid is large.

COUGH (Tussis)

Cough is only a symptom, but at times it may be so prominent a one as to appear to demand exclusive attention. The act of coughing is one of forcible or violent expiration, and may be caused by irritation of the mucous membrance, of the air-passages, inhalation of dust, derangement of the stomach, etc.

Treatment—In all cases coming on immediately after exposure to cold it is advisable to administer *Acon.* every two or three hours, or oftener, until relief is obtained, or until it is found to fail in bringing about improvement. Cough being often the first and only expression of congestion of the mucous membrance of the air-passages, is best treated, as is the affection itself, with this medicine. After *Acon.* the action of other remedies is more prompt and decided.

Indications for Treatment

Aconitum—Hard, dry, irritative cough, with fever; after exposure to cold.

---

* See Glossary.

Aralia—Night cough, coming on after the first sleep.

Ant.-Tart.—Loose cough, sputa copious, great weakness, vomiting.

Bryonia—Dry cough, with pain in chest, yellow phlegm.

Cina.—Dry or loose cough of a chronic character, when the child is suffering from Worms.

Drosera—Spasmodic cough, worse at night; second state of Whoopping-cough.

Hyoscyamus—Dry cough, worse on lying down at night.

Ipecac—Spasmodic cough with mucous expectoration, and tedency to Vomiting.

Phosph.—Hoarse cough, pain under breast-bone, rusty-coloured phlegm.

Pulsatilla—Loose cough, worse at night.

Spongia—Dry, hard, barking cough, hoarseness, burning or tickling in the windpipe.

Accessories—The diet should be light and given in small quantities, particularly if there be fever. A cold sponge-bath every morning, and frequent out-door exercise will often overcome a susceptibility to this affection. A good draught of cold water taken in the morning, and also on retiring, is both preventive and curative of cough, Lastly, children should be intrusted to make direct voluntary efforts to restrain the frequency and violence of coughing; for the result of such efforts will be found greatly to mitigate this symptom.

See also the Section on "Whooping-cough," "Pleurisy," "Bronchitis," "Inflammation of the Lungs," and "Croup" (page 61 and 111-124).

Chapter VI

DISEASES OF THE DIGESTIVE SYSTEM

TONGUE-TIE (Lingua Frenata)

On the under surface of the tongue there is a fold of tissue-like mucous membrane, called the *fraenum linguae*, which connects the contue with the floor of the mouth. Congetial *Tongue-tie* is said to exist when the attachment of the *fraenum* extends along the whole under-surface of the tongue to its tip. But this condition is extremely rare, and, even, when it exists, seldom given rise to any real inconvenience. The difficulty of speech with which it is sometimes associated proceeds from deeper causes, involving the brain and mind. When, however, the attachment of the *fraenum* is very thick and extensive, it may form a mechanical obstacle to sucking, and, later, to clear articulation. When, therefore, any difficulty of sucking exists, the state of the *fraenum linguae* should be examined, and, if necessary, divided. The little operation may be performed as follows. The infant should bemade to cry, by which act the *fraenum* will be fully exposed; then the doctor by means of a pair of round-ended scissors, keeping the points towards the back of the mouth, will make a very light notch. The backward direction on the scissors, and the small extent of the snip, are necessary to avoid wounding the artery of the *fraenum*, an accident that might give rise to serious haemorrhage.

INFLAMMATION OF THE MOUTH (Stomatitis)

Symptom—Heat, redness, dryness, and ulceration of the mucous membrane of the mouth; slight swelling and pain of the tongue, cheeks, gums, and palate; foetid breath, and salivation may also be present.

Treatment—This disease is most frequently amenable to the action of *Kali Choloricum*, but other remedies are sometimes called for. A dose of the medicine should be given three times a day.

Indications for the above and other Remedies

Hydrastis—Swelling, dark redness, and soreness of the tongue, gums, and cheek; ulceration of the lips and tongue; tenacious mucous in the mouth.

Kali Chlor.—Great soreness, foetid breath, and ulceration; especially after the allopathic use of *Mercury*.

Mercurius Sol. 3x—Slight cases; foetid breath, and an abudant flow of watery saliva.

Accessories—The mouth should be moistened frequently with thin barely-water, or with glycerine-and-water (one teaspoonful of glycerine to a large wineglass of water).

CANCRUM ORIS (Gangrenous Stomatitis)

Definition—A sloughing or gangrenous ulcer of the mouth, occasionally occurring in ill-fed children from two to six years old, residing in low, damp situations, or living in overcrowded rooms and breathing impure air.

Symptoms—The inflammation generally begins at the edges of the gums opposite the incisors of the lower jaw; the gums are white and spongy, and separate from the teeth, as if *Mercury* had produced its specific effects. Ulceration begins and extends along the gums until the jaws are implicated; and as the disease advances, the cheeks and lips swell, and form a tense indurated tumefaction. The teeth are apt to fall out; and the breath to become intolerably foetid, from a gangernous condition. There is generally enlargement and tenderness of the submaxillary glands. In severe forms of the disease, the destructive process rapidly extends, so that in a few days the lips, cheeks, tonsils, palate, tongue, and even half the face may become gangrenous, the teeth falling from their sockets, a horribly foetid saliva and fluid flowing from the parts.

Treatment—*Mercurius* is generally the specific for this affection. A dose may be administered three or four times a day. Next to *Mercurius, Mur.-Ac.* has been found most efficatious.

Indications for the above and other Remedies

Ars.—Extensive disorganizations of the mouth, extreme prostration.

Merc.-Sol. 3x—The most useful remedy; will rarely fail to prove efficacious, if the disease has not been cuased by any preparation of *Mercury*.

Mur.-Ac.—When the disease is associated with other diseases, such as Measles, Pneumonia, etc.

Sulph.-Ac.—Rapid spread of ulceration.

Sulph.—In chronic cases.

Accessories—The gums, teeth, and mouth should be frequently cleansed with a mixture of Condy's fluid one part, and water one hundred parts, or a weak lotion of carbolic acid and water (about ten drops of the former to a tumbler of the latter). Strong beef-tea, raw eggs beaten up in milk, and occasionally wine, are generally necessary.

SORE THROAT

Definition—Acute simple inflammation of the throat, including Simple Tonsillitis, Follicular Tonsillitis, and Acute Phyrangitis. The usual sore throat is generally either a Simple or a Follicular Tonsillitis, which may be accompanied by more or less Pharyngitis.

Symptoms—In Simple Acute Tonsillitis, one or both tonsils become deep red and swollen and are the seat of pain, more or less severe, usually much aggravated by swallowing. In Follicular Tonsillitis, in addition to these symptoms, the tonsils are sutdded with whitish-yellow spots, which are the orifices of the tonsillar crypts choked up with products of exudation. Both forms are accompanied by fever the temperature running up to 103° or 104°.

Cause—The real cause is microbic. Exciting causes are chill; bad hygienic surroundings, especially defective drainage. Tonsillitis is often part and parcel of a rheumatic infection in children; this is most improtant to remember. For the diagnosis from Diphtheria see page 57.

Treatment—*Aconite* should be given at once—a dose

every two hours. If it does not act favourably in a few hours, *Belladonna* will probably be called for.

Indications for the above and other Remedies

Aconitum—Dryness, roughness, and heat in the throat, with a choking sensation, hoarseness, fever.

Belladonna—Bright-red throat, feeling as if scraped raw with pain on swallowing.

Dulcamara—If from getting wet, or from damp, foggy air.

Mercurius Sol.—Sensation as of a lump in throat, worse at night, increased flow or saliva, white or yellow spots on throat.

Accessories—Hot fomentations round the neck; steaming the throat over a jug of boiling water containing a teaspoonful of Friar's balsam.

QUINSY (Suppurative Tonsillitis)

Definition—A suppurative inflammation of the tonsils, in which the inflammation and abscess tend to spread on to the soft palate.

Symptoms—Swelling of tonsils, severe throbbing pain, hoarseness, difficult swallowing and expectoration, Headache, pain in the back and limbs, foul tongue, offensive breath, shivering, high temperature (104° or 105°), and profound prostration, treminating in resolution or suppuration, or chronic enlargement.

Causes—As for "Sore Throat" (page 129).

Treatment—If seen very early the patient should have a few doses of *Aconitum*, followed by *Baryta Carb*. If suppuration be inevitable, *Hepar S.* should be administered. In some acute cases *Guaiacum* has been eminently successful in checking the progress of the disease. *Gunpowder* is also worth a trial.

Indications for the above and other Remedies

Aconitum—Pricking sensation in the throat, with much fever.

Belladonna—Redness and rawness of the throat, flushed face, glistening of the face, Headache.

Baryta Carb.—If given early in acute cases it is often very efficacious. Is very useful also in chronic cases.

Calc.-Carb.—Chronic cases in scrofulous persons.

Hepar S.—When suppuration has taken place.

Guaiacum—In cases accompanied with pains of a rheumatic neuralgic character.

Lycopodium—Ulceration and suppuation of tonsils, beginning on right side. Worse from 4 to 8 p.m.

Accessories—As for "Sore Throat" (page 130). As soon as it is certain that pus has formed, the abscess should be lanced.

Mercur.-Iod.—Considerable swelling, copious salivation, swelling of tongue, foetid breath.

CHRONIC TONSILLITIS ("Tonsils and Adenoids")

Definition—A chronic enlargement of the tonsils, in which there may be little evidence of active inflammation, accompanied by lymphoid masses in the naso-pharynx (an exaggeration of the so-called "pharyngeal tonsil").

Causation—In this condition cause and effect are much mixed up. Cold or Simple Nasal or Naso-pharyngeal Catarrh, by inducing a habit of mouth-breathing, leads to imperfect development of the nasal cavities and accessory sinuses, and this is believed to be a cause of adenoids. On the other hand adenoids undoubtedly themselves lead to a Chronic Naso-pharyngeal Catarrh and repeated cold-catching, with their natural result of chronic mouth-breathing. The want of hard food in the child's diet and consequent failure to exercise the jaws and muscles of mastication also lead to imperfect development of the naso-pharynx and the accessory sinuses and so to adenoids. The same is true of insufficient vitamins in the food. There is, however, without doubt a condition of *Congenital Adenoids,* in which an infant is born with an overgrowth of the lymphoid tissue normally found in the naso-pharynx. Hypertrophy of the lymphoid tissue of the tonsils is generally a concomitant of adenoids.

Symptoms—Mouth-breathing, snoring at night, nasal speech, impairment of smell and taste, nocturnal incontinence, the adenoidal facies (pinched-in nostrils, open mouth, vacant expression), fetor of the breath, earache and deafness (due to extension of catarrh to the Eustachian tube), enlarged cervical glands, paroxysmal cough, Bronchial Catarrh, backwardness, Asthma, Dyspepsia (from swallowing the mucus secreted by the adenoids), mental dulness, certain deformities of the chest (notably the "funnel breast"), a tendency to attacks of Acute Follicular Tonsillitis, a diminished resistance to such serious throat trouble as Diphtheria, and reflexly at times Convulsions and Laryngismus Stridulus. In congenital cases the chief symptoms are the nasal discharge, the snoring respiration, and the difficulty in taking the breast. Many remote troubles, as e.g. Arthritis, are traced to latent and smouldering foci of infection deep in the crypts of unhealthy tonsils.

Treatment—Congenital Adenoids, inasmuch as they interfere with taking the breast and with swallowing milk and so retard nutrition at a critical age, ought to be removed by operation. In acquired adenoids a trial may be made of homoeopathically chosen remedies (see below), of systematic deep-breathing exercises, of a nasal toilet (Hutchison recommends a solution of borax, one drachm to the pint, injected up the nostrils and allowed to run out by the mouth), and of painting the tonsils with a paint consisting of one part of tincture of iodine and seven parts of anaesthetic ether. By the age of about five, if marked improvement has not resulted (and earlier still if deafness threatens or Asthma or Convulsions occur), an operation should be undertaken for the removal of the adenoids and for extirpation of the tonsils by one of the modern complete methods. Such opertions ought always to be followed up by systematic education in nose-breathing by day and by the use at night, if necessary, of an elastic chinstrap to keep the lower jaw from dropping.

Indications for Homoeopathic Remedies

Baryta Carb.—Swollen tonsils. Quinsy. Children backward physically and mentally. Enlarged glands in neck.

Baryta Mur.—Similar to *Baryta Carb.*

Calc.-Carb.—Fat flabby children, very chilly, chalky complexion, sweating head, enlarged glands, readily catch cold.

Calc.-Phos.—Swollen tonsils and adenoids. Pale wasted children, chilly and readily catching cold. Bone troubles. Swollen glands.

Calc.-Iod.—Similar to Calc.-Phos.

Lycopod—Swelling and suppuration of tonsils beginning on right side. Wizened children. Worse from 4 to 8 p.m. Craves everything warm.

Sulphur—Dry unhealthy skin. Complains of heat, burning,

itching. Aversion to washing. When well-chosen remedies
have failed.

Tuberculinum—Tuberculosis feared or suspected, or comes
of tuberculous stock. Readily catches cold. When well-chosen
remedies have failed.

THRUSH—SORE MOUTH (Parasitic Stomatitis)

Definition—An inflammatory product, consisting of
white patches, on the lining membrane of the mouth and
throat. The white patches are now known to be a microscopic
parastic plant—the *Oidium albicans*—the sporules of which
increase with great rapidity, and form tubular fibrils. There is
also an increased formation of epithelial scales. The unhealthy
secretions of the mouth, particularly when *acid*, form a *nidus*
or breeding-ground for the vegetation.

Cases—Improper diet; unsuitable quality or quantity of
food given to infants fed with the bottle or spoon, neglect of
general cleanliness (especially dirty bottles, teats, etc.), also
neglecting to wipe out the baby's mouth after every feed, bad
drainage, etc. A scrofulous constitution may operate as a
predisposing cause. The disease also occurs during the course
of Measles, Enteric fever, Diabetes, and Consumption; it is
then generally indicative of an early fatal termination.

Symptoms—There is generally some febrile disturbance;
the child is fretful, often refuses the breast on account of pain
experienced in sucking; there is usually vomiting, and a thin,
watery Diarrhoea, caused by deranged intestinal secretions.
The local symptoms consist of innumerable white specks, like
little bits of curd, which are sometimes so connected as to
form a continuous, dirty, diphtheritic-like covering over the
tongue, gums, palate, and inside of the cheeks and lips. In
severe cases, vegetations line the whole interior of the mouth,

and extend even to the fauces and down the gullet; the buttocks also become red and excoriated by the acid secretions; the parastic plants, however, are not developed on the interior of the stomach or bowels, but are restricted to thsoe portions of the mucous tract which are studded with scaly epithelium.

Prognosis—In children otherwise strong, thrush, which is caused by improper food or want of cleanliness, may be readily cured by one or more of the following remedies, and by correction of the faulty hygienic condition. If it occurs as a complication in the course of an exhausting disease, or after a lengthened course of improper food, in which the digestion and assimilation of nourishment must be necessarily imperfect, the prospect of recovery becomes proportionately diminished. Diarrhoea, too, is by no means infrequent, especially in feeble children, and increases the gravity of the case.

Treatment—*Borax* and *Mercurius* are the chief remedies for this disease. The latter is perhaps more often employed than the former. The medicine selected should be given three times a day.

Indications for the above and other Remedies

Arsenicum—Dark colour of the patches; offensive odour from the mouth; severe Diarrhoea and great constitutional prostration.

Borax—Child's rest is much disturbed, salivation, the aphthae bleed freely.

Mercurius Sol.—Dribbling saliva, offensive breath, Diarrhoea; if administered when the white specks first appears, it is often alone sufficient.

Sulphur—In convalescence, and when there are eruptions on the skin.

Accessories—The child's mouth should be washed with a weak solution of *Borax* (ten grains to one ounce of water), or bicarbonate of soda (a drachm in half a pint of water), by means of a soft brush, two or three times a day. Before using the lotion the mouth should be well cleansed with a piece of linen rag squeezed out of warm water.

A point of first consideration is *suitable diet*. If Thrush be distinctly traceable to any disease in the mother which cannot be quickly cured, the infant should be at once provided with a wet-nurse, or weaned, and fed as directed in page 20.

Prevention—Every variety of strach-food is unsuitable for an infant. Diet is to be as prescribed in page 20. Strict cleanliness is particularly necessary. After each meal the mouth should be washed, to prevent the accumulation of milk about the gums. This simple measure will often prevent the appearance of Thrush. In like manner, the mother's nipple should be cleansed each time after giving it to the infant. Well-ventilated rooms, and abundance of out-of-door air, every day, in suitable weather, will prove of extreme value, rendering the secretions more healthy, and raising the tone of the general system.

DISORDERS OF DENTITION

To enable our readers to recognize the disorders of Dentition (in itself a natural process), we shall briefly sketch the progress of healthy teething. There are two sets of teeth: the first—the milk teeth—appears during the first two years of life, and falls out about the seventh or eight year. As the first set falls out it is replaced by the permanent, which is not completed till adult life.

The milk teeth generally appear in the following order:—
About the sixth month the two middle incisors of the lower
jaw, followed in a few weeks by the corresponding incisors of
the upper jaw; next appear the two outside incisors of the
lower jaw; and soon after those of the upper; after another
interval of perhaps about two months, the first four molars,
then the eye-teeth, and, lastly, four other molars, completing
by about the second year, the teeth of the first set. Should
there be any little deviation from this order, or should
Dentition be a little prolonged, no great importance need be
attached to it.

Although Dentition is a natural process of development in
many children it is a trying one, and may even call into fatal
activity latent tendencies to disease. Indeed, in the Registrar-
General's annual report for 1884 no less than 4,942 deaths are
ascribed to this cause. In consequence of the increased activity
and excitement in the vascular system, combined with the
nervous irritation which sometimes attends Dentition, local or
constitutional disturbances are likely to arise in delicate
children. Rickets, for example, greatly influences the progress
of teething. If this disease sets in previously to the
commencement of Dentition, the evolution of the teeth may
be almost indefinitely delayed; or if some are already cut,
further progress may be arrested. Rickety children of eighteen
months or two years old may often be seen with very few
teeth, and those few black and carious.

Symptoms—Bronchitis; restlessness, starting, as if in
fright, or interrupted sleep; sudden occurrence of febrile
symptoms; hot, swollen, or tender gums, and increased flow
of saliva; derangement of the digestive organs—sickness,
Diarrhoea, or Constipation; and sometimes Spasms and
Convulsions. Diarrhoea and other symptoms of Indigestion
are most frequent in the summer and autumn, and when,
therefore, children are not exposed to sudden changes.

Causes—Rickets and general delicacy. The exciting causes are *irregular feeding; excessive feeding; improper quality* of food, and deficiency of vitamins. Disordered Dentition is often coincident with a change of diet from the mother's milk to various articles which are unsuited to the age of the child. Inflammatory affection of the gums, or disproportion between the jaw and the number and form of the teeth, are also causes of suffering. (See the next Section.)

Treatment—*Chamomilla* is an excellent medicine for most cases of disordered Dentition, and, in the absence of fever, should be considered. It may be given every two or three hours.

Indications for the several Remedies

Aconitum—Feverishness, restlessness, inflamed gums.

Calc.-Carb.—Cases complicated with slimy Diarrhoea; in scrofulous patients.

Chamomilla—Bilious purging, intestinal irritation, cough, nervousness, and fretfulness.

Kreasotum—In cachectic children; agitation and wakefulness; gums inflamed; Constipation; teeth decay as soon as they appear.

Additional Remedies

Arsen. (with much emaciation); *Bell.* (flushed face, nervous irritability); *Merc.-Sol.* (green or bloody motions); *Podoph.* (pain in paroxysms, with Prolapsus Ani); *Sil.* (much perspiration about the head when falling asleep).

Accessory Treatment—*Regularity in the times of feeding and sleep;* correction of any habits in the mother which may affect the child unfavourably; restriction to *suitable quantities* of food at one time. (See "Diet," page 20-25.) *Keeping the feet warm, and allowing the child to be much in the open air.*

DECAY OF THE TEETH

The function of the teeth is so important that it is impossible to over-estimate the necessity of exercising due care in their management during the whole period of childhood. A good set of teeth is one of the best guarntees a child can possess of good digestion and prolonged health; and this blessing it is generally possible to attain by the exercise of early care. A large proportion of the patients who come under our observation, including persons of all ages, suffer from a more or less deteriorated state of the teeth and gums. Our opportunities of investigating this subject have been extensive, for it is one of the points upon which we make definite inquiry, more especially in cases of Indigestion and defective nutrition. Our own observations are confirmed by dentists of long practice, who have noticed the increasing prevalence of carious teeth.

Causes—The early decay of the teeth is due, in a great measure, to preventible causes, the chief of which are the following:—

☞ *A Crowled State of the Teeth*—In some children the jaws are so small or irregular that there is not sufficient room for proper development. The consequence is that they overlap, and, pressing against each other, damage the enamel. Moreover in this condition there is greater probability than in a normal condition that particles of food will be retained in the mouth, and decomposing, the formation of caries will be favoured.*

☞ *Insufficient Use of the Teeth*—This is consequent on the kind of food taken, and on its preparation. The prevalent use of sops and of soft new bread is productive of much evil. Nothing is more suitable for a child, with the incisors cut, than a crust of stale bread, or a bone, on which to exercise and harden the teeth and gums. The result of insufficient use of the teeth is that the jaws are imperfectly developed, the gums become soft and spongy, the teeth grow irregularly, are easily loosened, and drop out. For it is with the teeth as with all other organs and functions of the body, the less they are employed for the purposes to which they are assigned, the more rapidly they become enfeebled and degenerate. Resistance gives strength. The resistance of tough food affords that healthy pressure which promotes circulation in the vessels, gives fixedness to the teeth, and necessitates the formation of that hard texture which wears well even when the enamel is gone.

☞ *Constitutional Debility*—Whatever enfeebles the general system enfeebles every part of it. If the standard of health be lowered by disregard of hygienic measures, or in any other manner, the teeth will suffer; they will decay for want of sufficient nutrition.

Indications for Treatment

Kreasotum—Sour state of the secretions of the mouth and stomach, with *frequent vomiting;* soreness of the gums.

---

* The first teeth should be preserved as long as possible, and when decayed should, unless too far gone, be filled. Extraction of the first teeth leads to contraction of the jaws, and consequent trouble with the second set.

Mercurius Sol. 6—Looseness of the teeth; retraction and bleeding of the gums; *excessive flow of saliva;* foetid breath.

Silicea—Soft, crumbly state of the teeth, associated with symptoms of *Rickets.*

Staphysagria—*Blackness* of the teeth; paleness, swelling, soreness, and erosion of the gums; looseness of the teeth.

Preventive Treatment—This may be inferred from the causes already mentioned. To prevent the crowding of the teeth, an experienced and skilful dentist should be consulted, who will remove superfluous teeth, selecting for extraction any that may be hopelessly decayed, or those which are most liable to early degeneracy, viz., the first permanent molars. We have repeatedly advised this course, with the most satisfactory results. Personal appearance has been improved by the greater regularity of the teeth; for the vacancies occasioned by removals have been quickly filled by the adjustment of the teeth to the vacant spaces. To prevent deterioration, we recommend a return to the primitive custom of eating *whole meal bread.* It gives the healthy stimulus which the teeth and gums require; it is more nutritious to the system; and it supplies in considerable quantity the silica and phosphates from which enamel and dentine are formed. We also advise parents to allow the children the vulgar gratification of nibbling a bone now and then. Sweets should only be allowed in moderation; strong acids, some of the preparations of iron, and hot drinks are always prejudicial. Cleanliness is essential to the prevention of decay. The bristles of the tooth-brush should be moderately soft, and not too thickly set. Where food is liable to become entangled between the teeth, the brush should be used after every meal. Not only animal food, but particles of white bread originate degenerative changes, and should be removed. Tooth-powder is unnecessary except after the teeth have been neglected; it may then be requuired for a short time to remove carious incursation. In any case the tooth-powder should not be harsh or medicated. Such as feels rough and gritty when rubbed between the thumb and finger should not be used, as it will scratch and injure the enamel. Brushing with simple water should be commenced directly when the teeth appear. An apple last thing at night is excellent for cleaning the teeth. Finally, vitamins in abundance in the food (as in butter, dripping, brown bread, fresh fruit, and greens), food well masticated, plenty of fresh air inhaled through the nose, will result in well-formed jaws, good teeth, and no adenoids.

TOOTHACHE (Odontalgia)

Toothache is often a distressing ailment of childhood, and is far from being uncommon, especially during the decay of the first teeth. The most frequent exciting *cuases* are sudden changes of temperature, general ill-health, and irritation of the bared nerve by particles of food.

Indications for Treatment

Aconitum—Toothache brought on by *cold,* or accompanied by *fever symptoms.*

Arsenicum—*Intermittent* toothache; burning or cutting pains; general *prostration.*

Belladonna—*Pain,* extending to the *temples,* particularly the right: *redness of the face, burning, throbbing,* and heat of the head.

Bryonia—Pain aggravated by *hot or cold food;* the cheek being tender to the touch.

Chamomilla—*Unbearable paroxysms* of pain; nightly aggravation: redness of one cheek and paleness of the other.

Mercurius Sol. 6—Pain starting from loose or *decayed teeth,* occurring in the night, accompanied with perspiration that gives no relief; pain *extending to the ears;* gumboil.

Kreasotum—This is a valuable remedy when *caries* exist, with red and painful gums, *offensive breath,* etc.

Pulsatilla—Pain *from indigestible food,* fat, pastry, etc., pain on the *left* side of the face.

Staphysagria—Toothache in *blackened,* decayed teeth; the teeth feel too long.

Accessory Treatment—The application of heat will sometimes give relief; in other cases, when the temple throbs, a small stream of cold water eases the pain. The digestive organs should be brought into a healthy condition, the action of the bowels should be regulated, and very hot or very cold food avoided.

Electricity frequently gives speedy relief. Using a constant current of eight or ten elements, the negative pole is applied to the cheek near the aching tooth, and the positive pole to the back of the neck. Improvement ensues in a few minutes.

In some cases the only remedy is *extraction*, especially if the tooth be loose, much decayed, and unfit for mastication; but in most cased the pain may be relieved by homoeopathic remedies. If the pain be in the parmanent teeth, and the caries be recent and slight, the decayed portion may frequently be removed, the cavity filled with a suitable material, and thus preserved a useful member for years. A qualified dentist should be consulted. (See also the previous Section).

ACUTE DYSPEPSIA (Acute Gastric Catarrh)

Symptoms—Sudden onset; nausea and Vomiting; furred tongue; prostration; often a high temperature.

Causes—Irritating food and chill whether from cold air or cold bathing. (These often produce in addition an acute intestinal Catarrh, manifested by Diarrhoea.)

The patient is liable to recurrent attacks of a milder Dyspepsia, in which there is less but longer lasting fever, furred tongue, some vomiting, and often Diarrhoea as well.

Indications for Treatment

Antimonium Crudum—*Thickly-furred, white tongue;* great thirst; painfulness of the stomach to pressure; nausea; *eructions;* poor appetite; vomiting of bile, with Diarrhoea.

Ipecacuanha—Aversion to food and *vomiting* of *mucous.* This is especially suitable when the breast-milk disagrees with a child, and is returned.

Nux Vomica—Aversion to food and drink; the matters vomited are sour or foetid; vomiting of green bilious matter; *Constipation.*

Pulsatilla—Simple vomiting *from indigestible food;* or when due to debility of the stomach.

Accessory Treatment—Child must be kept in bed on a restricted diet. If vomiting is severe and urgent, nothing should be given but sips of iced water or of very hot water. If it is a first attack, it should be remembered that these symptoms of Acute Gastric Catarrh may represent Appendicitis or the initial stage of some such acute specific disease as Pneumonia or Meningitis. With recurrent so-called "bilious" attacks the strong possibility of a relapsing Appendicitis should be borne in mind.

CHRONIC (or Habitual) VOMITING

Chronic Vomiting in *infants* is most often due to errors in diet. These are to be corrected in accordance with the instructions under Sections on pages 40-42. It may also be due to narrowing of the pyloric orifice of the stomach (so-called "congenital" pyloric stenosis). Here the vomiting does not begin till ten days or a fortnight after birth and therefore is not congenital; the narrowing is probably due to spasm of uncertain origin. The manifestations of this condition are extremely forcible ("projectile") vomiting of food and mucus, with Constipation, emaciation, and visible gastric peristalsis (waves of muscular contraction passing along the stomach). This is a condition for the physician first of all. Hutchison recommends washing out the stomach once or twice a day with weak solution of bicarbonate of soda, and giving the breast (or failing that, peptonized milk diluted with an equal quantity of water) frequently and in small quantities—it may be every half hour or every hour or at longer intervals. Internally; try *Nux Vomica, Bismuthum, Cuprum Ars.*, and *Mag.-Phos.* in that order. If after a fortnight of this treatment there is no definite improvement, operation ought probably to be resorted to.

Chronic Vomiting in *older children* takes several forms. It may be simply due to recurring Gastritis, very similar to the acute Gastric Catarrh described on page 143, and to be treated in much the same way. (Remember, however, that this so-called recurring Gastritis is often really a manifestation of a chronic relapsing Appendicitis, for which the only safe treatment is operation.) It may be the leading feature of recurring "bilious" attacks, which, when not due to Appendicitis, are often really a kind of nerve-storms, coming on in nervous children, especially under strain of excitement or fatigue. They are often accompanied by a slight rise of temperature. The treatment is simple—bed, starvation for twelve or twenty-four hours, and *Ignatia*. There is a form of "bilious" attack in which in addition to Vomiting there is Constipation, dry furred tongue, a sweetish heavy breath, and drowsiness and slight fever. There is acetone in the urine. This acidosis or acid-intoxication (which accounts for the sweetish breath and is similar to what is observed in serious or terminal

Diabetes) may, if not promptly neutralized by alkalies, prove fatal. "The main indication is to give bicarbonate of soda freely to counteract the acidosis. It may be given by the mouth *ad lib.*, dissolved in water, and though much will be vomited, some is retained" (Hutchison). What is the cause of this kind of attack is not certainly knwon, but it appears to have something to do with an excess of fat or sugar or both in the diet. such patients should have their milky, fatty, an sugary food drastically reduced.

In these types of chronic Vomiting there is usually good health between the attacks. But in what Eustace Smith called "mucous disease" (really a chronic Gstro-Intestinal Catarrh (see page 150)), the symptoms are persistent and continuous.

Indications for Treatment

Arsenicum—Dryness of the mouth, with bitter taste and disagreeable odour; Thrush; ulcerated, coated, or *cracked tongue;* Vomiting after food of watery fluid; great tenderness and Colic; *prostration and emaciation;* watery Diarrhoea.

Calc.-Carb.—Chronic Vomiting, with *swelling and hardness of bowels,* and constipated or offensive motions. Very suitable to small or weakly children.

Graphites—Vomiting, great flatulence, Constipation of knotty stools covered with mucus.

Hydrastis—Vomiting of ropy mucus, Constipation without desire for stool, ropy Naso-pharyngeal Catarrh.

Kreasotum—A poor constitution, general ill-health, and *persistent Vomiting.*

Nux Vomica—This is an excellent remedy in some forms of *Chronic Vomiting.*

Pulsatilla—Tongue covered with whitish mucus; vomiting of mucus or bile; mucous *Diarrhoea.* Most useful for fair children with blue eyes.

Veraturm Alb.—Excessive Vomiting, especially with *watery, nocturnal,* or *involuntary Diarrhoea;* slow pulse; faintness; *coldness of the face, tongue, and extremities.*

ACUTE INFANTILE DIARRHOEA.

The frequency of Dioarrhoea in early childhood, especially during Dentition and its large contribution to infantile mortality, especially in summer and autumn, and the fact that it depends mainly on obvious and removable causes, render the due consideration of the subject of great importance.

Varieties—Diarrhoea in childhood may be of varying degrees of severity, ranging from a simple passing looseness having no constitutional effects (*simple or catarrhal Diarrhoea*) up to *acute epidemic Diarrhoea,* which, having grave constitutional effects and being attended with a high mortality, is here more particularly considered. In any case remedies will be chose from the same list, due regard being paid to the severity of the case.

Causes—Epidemic Diarrhoea of children comes on chiefly in summer, and the hotter the summer the more prevalent and virulent is the disease. "It is when the thermometer, immersed four feet in the soil, begins to record a temperature of about 56° F. that epidemic Diarrhoea becomes most common" (Hutchison). The disease is microbic, and infection is encouraged by every kind of bad sanitation and by chill. The microbes are actually conveyed in the milk. Minor forms of Diarrhoea (as e.g. in *Coeliac Disease,* see page 82, and in Eustace Smith's *Mucous Disease,* see page 150), are often associated with an excess of starchy or sugary food. The dietetic remedy for these is obvious. But the severer forms are due to milk infection.

Symptoms—These vary extremely, even in recent and acute attacks, from a slight, painless increase in the quantity, frequency, and altered consistence of the normal evacuations, to violent, painful, and frequent purging; liquid evacuations, perhaps several times every hour, being ejected with spasmodic force. In the latter cases the motions are green or spinach-like, resembling those produced by administration of *Mercury*, but assume a yellow appearance during recovery. Frequently they contain the casein of undigested milk in the form of numerous white specks. In the more severe stage, they are sometimes streaked with blood, and mixed with mucus. There is also generally sickness, thirst, and an interruption in the nutritive processes. Acute Diarrhoea rapidly reduces the firmness of the muscles, and if the drain be severe, in two or three days there is a marked loss of flesh and strength. The eyes are sunken, the features pinched and livid; the pulse rapid, feeble, and nearly imperceptible; and the extremities cold and shrunken. On the other hand, after the cessation of an acute attack, the lost flesh and vigour are quickly regained, and the child soon recovers his wonted colour and spirits.

Indications for Treatment

Arsenicum—Neglected or advanced cases, in which there is aggravation at night, and *unquenchable thirst;* when the various measures employed seem useless, and the *pale, sunken face* gives evidence that the disease is making serious inroads, *Ars.* often succeeds. But it is more often required in *chronic* than in acute Diarrhoea.

Chamomilla—Diarrhoea during *Dentition*, or from *cold*, with *fretfulness* or restlessness; colicky pains; greenish, watery. forthy, and offensive evacuations; yellowness of the whites-of-the-eyes, and sallow skin.

Ipecacuanha—Simple Diarrhoea, with straining or blood-streaked motions, from overloading the stomach, or during hot weather with *sickness*, the latter symptoms being more marked than the Diarrhoea.

Iris.—Bilious evacuations, with sickness; *Cholera Infantum*, especially when *Vomiting* is frequent.

Mercurius Corr.—Evacuation containing *blood*, and passed with *excessive straining*.

Mercurius Dulcis—Stools green, whitish *clay-coloured*, watery, or mixed with mucus; *straining*, nausea, and thirst.

Podophyllum—Profuse, *sudden*, foetid, exhausting discharges, *worse in the morning* and forenoon; frequent retching without vomiting; drowsiness; rolling and perspiration of the head; moaning and restlessness; *Diarrhoea better at night*.

Veratrum Allum.—*Choleraic* Diarrhoea, with frequent, copious, *watery discharges*, occurring in *gushes*, and accompanied by excessive *Vomiting* and *prostration;* spasmodic drawing up the legs, *cold sweat* on the forehead, and *coldness of the abdomen*. This remedy is often valuable after others have been uselessly administerd.

China—Loose foetid stools, with copious discharge of foetid flatus, preceded by painful Colic.

Phos.—Painless profuse Diarrhoea, "pouring away as from a hydrant"; vomiting of what has been drunk as soon as it becomes warm in the stomach.

Accessory Treatment—In epidemic Diarrhoea the great thing is to withhold milk. Indeed in any Diarrhoea a child may for a time require no food but boiled water or albumin-water (white of egg in water), or some thin meat broth. Water it should have in plenty, and it should be kept warm in bed. As the child gets better, return may be made to normal diet *via* whey, and after whey milk and water in varying proportions, the milk, if necessary, being peptonized and the water always boiled.

If these instructions are followed and remedies given according to their homoeopathic indications, the elaborate ritual recommended by some of washing out both stomach and rectum will hardly ever be necessary.

Virulent cases which in spite of every measure have come to the verge of collapse or which have not come under treatment until far gone, will require the hot mustard bath and an injection under the skin of the flank of a few ounces of boiled normal saline solution (a teaspoonful of common salt to the pint), which may be given three times a day.

CHRONIC GASTRO-INTESTINAL CATARRH
("Mucous Disease")

Definition—This is a Dyspepsia of the second Dentition and one of the wasting diseases of childhood. Its importance lies, first, in the fact that it is quite common and if untreated or inadequately treated, very chronic; and secondly, in its liability to be mistaken for Tuberculosis. It is important in cases of this sort to take, and keep a record of, the temperature. A persistent slight temperature would point to Tuberculosis. "Mucous Disease" (as Eustace Smith called it), however, predisposes to Tuberculosis. (See "Tuberculous Ulceration of Bowel," page 80).

Symptoms—Vomiting; pain and flatulence after food; Diarrhoea, often the pale pasty motions, often "lienteric" (i.e. coming on immediately after, or even during, a meal), often alternating with the passage of constipated mucus-coated lumps; appetite capricious, sometimes poor, sometimes ravenous, sometimes for unnatural articles such as coal and chalk; furred tongue; progressive wasting; languor and irritability; pallor of the face; disturbed, restless sleep, often accompanied by incontinence of urine; and lastly evidence of "tonsils and adenoids" at one end and "worms" at the other.

Causation—Possibly an inherrent defect of asimilating power. Whatever the essential cause is, a main exciting cause is sugar and starch in the diet; where the stools are pale it may be inferred that the milk is not properly digested. Whether the "tonsils and adenoids" stand in a causal relation to the "Mucous Disease" or are themselves caused by it, is not easy to say. The worms undoubtedly are due to the unhealthy condition of the bowel.

Indications for Treatment

Arsenicum—Bluish or white tongue; *excessive, unquenchable thirst*; Vomiting; distention of, and pain in, the abdomen; Diarrhoea worse after food, especially after midnight; motions watery, slimy, black, green, whitish, or blody, and *frequent* and *scanty*; *weakness and emaciation*; distressing restlessness, sleeplessness; pale face; coldness of the extremities.

Calcarea Carbonica—Diarrhoea in weakly, palefaced, emaciated, scrofulous children, who are liable to glandular swellings on taking the least cold; undigested, sour, papescent, frothy, foetid, or involuntary stools; thread-worms; pains during a motion, and faintness afterwards.

Carbo Vegetabilis—*Offensive Diarrhoea*; thirst afer a motion; much flatulence, acidity, and ill-humour.

Cina—Diarrhoea associated with worms; starting and crying out in sleep, and other worm symptoms.

China—Diarrhoea, worse after eating; yellow, watery, undigested, blackish, or putrid motions; flatulence; loss of appetite; debility.

Croton Tiglium—Thin, yellowish-brown, putrid evacuations, expelled suddenly, and induced by eating; involuntary stool during sleep.

Iodium—Thin, foetid evacuations, with distention of the

bowels; emaciation from unassimilated food; hectic symptoms. It is especially suited to the Diarrhoea of strumous children.

Mercurius Iodatus—Chronic Diarrhoea, with hardness and enlargement of the abdomen; the glands may sometimes be felt on pressing the hand upon the bowels, which impart a knotty feeling. This remedy is most suitable for the stunted and ill-nourished children of weakly parents, particularly when scrofulous enlargements or Abscesses exist.

Mercurius Sol.—Frequent evacuations of frothy mucus, or whitish, green, offensive, or bloody stools; excoriation of the anus; violent pain; Jaundice. If there is severe *straining,* with other dysenteric symptoms, *Merc.-Cor.* is preferable.

Phosphorus—Chronic Diarrhoea in children having a consumptive tendency; yellow tinge of the eyes and skin; great prostration; chest complications.

Accessory Treatment—What has been said under "Causation" indicates the chief non-medicinal line of treatment. The starch and the sugar in the diet must be severely restricted. The eating of "sweets" must be stopped. If the stools are pale, milk should be limited. Tepid abdominal compresses and general massage are useful. An abdominal belt of flannel is often efficacious. Children should be protected against atmospheric changes by warm clothing. Lastly, change of air is often necessary and prmptly curative. If no other end be served, it may remove the little patient out of the range of some undetected and unthought-of cause of the disease, which exists in the air or water.

APPENDICITIS

Definition—An infective inflamation of the appendix vermiformis of the caecum.

Symptoms—Pain and Colic, nausea and Vomiting, a temperature from 100°F. to 102° or 103°, and tenderness in the appendix region, that is round about McBurney's spot, which lies at the junction of the middle and outer thirds of a line joining the navel to the right anterior superior spine. The pain usually begins in the epigastric (stomach) or umbilical (navel) region, but after a little while shifts to, and becomes fixed in, the appendix region. Pain is the first symptom; Vomiting comes on soon afterwards. In the case of an appendix which hangs down into the pelvis, no tenderness may be elicited until a rectal examination is made. This should never be omitted. In the ordinary course the temperature after remaining up for three or four days gradually subsides, the pulse rate declining coincidently. A sudden drop of the temperature to normal is a bad sign, suggesting perforation or gangrene of the appendix. Decline of the temperature, accompanied by a steady rise of the pulse rate, is extremely ominous. But the temperature and pulse may both fall and the patient may lose his pain and say that he feels much better, and yet the appendix may at the same time be absolutely gangrenous. The course of a case of appendicitis is so incalculable, a paitent who has not seemed very ill may so rapidly reach death's door, that probably the only safe course is to operate as soon as the diagnosis is clear. The anxious, haggard countenance, board-like rigidity in the right groin, secondary Vomiting (Vomiting coming on again after it has stopped), indicate an infection of the peritoneum and call for immediate operation.

In Chronic Appendicitis there may be few if any localizing signs, there may be little or no appendicular tenderness, nothing in fact but somewhat vague indigestion symptoms— pain, sickness, flatulences, or symptoms which are often labelled "bilious"; but if the history is carefully investigated, it is generally possible to find that there has been at some time in the past and acute or subacute attack of Appendicitis. Recurring "bilious" attacks in a child or a chronic indigestion that does not yield to dieting and carefully chosen remedies should always be carefully scrutinized from the "appendix" point of view. The right treatment for chronic Appendicitis is operation; the "latent," "chronic" or "quiescent" appendix has been proved by abundant and most tragic experience to be no safer than a latent, chronic, or quiescent volcano.

Diagnosis—This is not always easy. The comonest mistake in the case of children is to mistake acutely inflamed glands, often tuberculous, in the appendix neighbourhood, for Appendicitis. No particular harm is done by operating on such cases; indeed, even when the glands are not removed, the patient are often curiously better for having daylight let into their abdomens.

Causes—The real cause is microbic. Exciting causes may be chill, excessive muscular strain, a heavy indigestible meal, etc.

Treatment

Belladonna and *Merc.-Cor.*—Should be used alternately every hour or every half hour according to urgency, pending the preparations for operation. Hot Fomentations should be applied to the abdomen. Where for any reason it is decided to postpone operations until the appendix is "quiescent," Silicea will often usefully follow up *Bell.* and *Merc.-Cor.*

PROLAPSUS ANI—FALLING OF THE BOWEL

Definition—A prostrusion of the mucous lining of the returm through the anal orifice, after the action of the bowel, which goes back of itself, or is easily replaced.

Causes—Long-continued Constipation of Diarrhoea; purgatives; straining excited by the irritation of worms, or of stone in the bladder; laxity and delicacy of constitution. Although not confined to them, it is most frequent in children.

Indications for Treatment

Arsenicum—When there are hot, loose motions preceded by colicky pains and thirst.

Calc-Carb.—In chronic cases in scrofulous children.

Lycopodium—Inflamed rectum, much flatulence in lower bowel.

Merc.-Cor.—Much tenesmus, with blood in stools.

Podphyllum—Prolapsus of the rectum; loose motions, of a brownish hue, hot, and having an acrid odour.

Accessories—When Prolapsus occurs after the action of the bowel, the protrusion should be reduced by placing the child across the lap, and making pressure on the protruded part with the fingers, previously lubricated, and carried beyond the contracting ring of the muscle around the anus. Prolapsus occasioned by straining from thread-worms is usually corrected by the treatment prescribed in the Section on Worms. Bathing the parts with cold water every morning, and injections of water, are useful.

The child should lie down for a short time after the action of the bowels. Constipation should be prevented by the measures elsewhere prescribed (page 158). The diet should be wholesome and unstimulating.

WORMS (Entozoa)

The worms that most commonly infest children are of three varieties—the thread-worm (Oxyuris vermicularis); the round-worm (Ascaris lumbricoides); and the tape-worm (Taenia mediocanellata). The first two are most common, the tape-worm being very rare in children under three years of age.

Thread-worms are from a third to half and inch in length, white and thread-like, moving rapidlay. They inhabit the rectum chiefly, often in very large numbers, and cause great irritation.

The round-worm is from six to fifteen inches long, similar to the comon earth-worm, but paler and thinner, It lives generally in the small intestines; but is sometimes passed upwards into the stomach and expelled by vomiting, or downwards, and ejected with the evacuations. It often exists in couples.

The tape-worm is white, flat, and jointed, varying in length from a few feet to several yards. It generally exists alone.

Symptoms—Thread-worms give rise to itching and irritation about the anus, especially troublesome in the evening; impaired or capricious appetite, offensive breath, picking at the nose, grinding of lthe teeth, straining at stool, falling of the bowel, Pruritus vulvae, disturbed sleep, general restlessness, and irritability.

When *Round-worms* exist in large numbers and get tangled up in a ball, there may be, in addition to the above symptoms, signs of intestinal obstruction, intermittent Diarrhoea, Convulsions, Chorea, etc. The round-worm may be dangerous from its habit of migrating. It may get into the larynx and cause fatal asphyxia.

The symptoms of *Tape-worm* are less marked; sensations of weight or gnawing in the abdomen; great appetite, and sometimes nausea and Diarrhoea.

Worms are frequently not suspected till seen in the evacuations.

Causes—The predisposing cause of worms is an unhealthy, *slimy* condition of the intestines of infants and young children, from improper feeding. When the conditions are fabourable for the development of worms, their germs or eggs, conveyed into the system by drinking impure water, by eating imperfectly-washed vegetables, or underdone meat, find a nest in which to grow and multiply.

Treatment—Where thread- or round-worms exist, *Cina* will usually the found an effective medicine. The tape-worm will require the oil of the male fern, sometimes in large doses, for its expulsion.

Indications for the several Remedies

Ant.-Curd.—White tongue, white mucous Diarrhoea.

Cina.—Boring at the nose; livid semicircles under the eyes; tossing about or suddenly *crying out in sleep;* nausea and Vomiting; griping, itching at the anus; *white, thick urine;* Epilepsy, Convulsions, or other nervous disorders.

Male Fern Oil—One of the most useful and reliable remedies in *Tape-worm.*

Mercurius Sol. 6—Whitish, greenish, pappy, or bloody evacuations, with tenesmus; distention of the abdomen; *foetid breath; great flow of saliva;* restlessness at night.

Sulphur—Worm-colic; *Constipation;* and to complete the cure.

Santonin 3x—Is good both for thread and roundworms.

Urtica Urens—Excessive *itching of the anus,* especially at night, from thread-worms.

Additional Remedies—*Ars., Calc.-C., Ignat., Puls., Santon., Teucrium.*

Accessories—When there is much irritation, a small injection of warm salt-and-water (a tablespoonful to half-a-pint) or an infusion of quassi may be used at bedtime, for several days. The application of a weak mercurial ointment to the anus at night relieves itching and prevents the worms from wandering. Hutchison recomends that the child should wear sleeping garments so constructed as to make access of the fingers to the anus impossible. F.H. Lorentz states that the thread-worm develops from ova only in the anal canal and that in his experience thorough washing of the anal region after every stool has been followed by excellent results.

For round-worm *Santonin* should be given after the bowel has been thoroughly empited.

For tape-worm it is best to keep the child in bed for two or three days on a very light, readily assimilable diet (milk, eggs, broth), the bowels being thoroughly empited. A dose of purgative having been given the night before, give male fern (*Filix Mas*) in capsules containing 15 grains every quarter of an hour for four doses. An hour later give half an ounce of mist. sennae co. The resulting motions should be passed into water, shaken up the filtered through black muslin, a search being made for the head, which is elongated and tapering, "a thin white filament about the size of a large pin." As long as the head cannot be found, there is liability to recurrence, but treatment should not be repeated for two months.

CONSTIPATION

Causes—Constipation in infants is almost invariably due to improper feeding, particularly the too early use of starchy kinds of food, which may occasion great mischief; irregularitis of diet in the mother of the sucking infant; purgatives, etc.

It may also be a symptom attendant on fever, disease of the liver or brain, etc., and and will then disappear with the derangement on which it depends, without special treatment.

Symptoms—Headache, feverishness, languor, irritability, restlessness, loss of appetite, distention of the abdomen, furred tongue, colic, frequent but inefficient urging to relieve the bowel, or the inclination may be altogether absent; disturbed sleep, etc. Vomiting is occasionally a symptom of obstinate Constipation. Remote results are Hernia and Prolapse of the Rectum.

Treatment—*Bryonia, Nux Vomica,* and *Sulphur* are the medicines which are most useful in Constipation. In all cases it is well to commence with *Sulphur.* A dose night and morning of the medicine will usually be sufficient.

Indications for the several Remedies

Bryonia—Large motions passed with difficulty; irritability; headache; brown tongue.

Lycopodium—Is especially useful when there is much flatulence in the lower bowel.

Mercurius Sol.—Sallow skin, the white-of-the eyes being yellowish; profuse secretion of saliva; pale, whitish motions.

Nux Vomica—Frequent ineffectual urging, restless sleep, irritability.

Opium—Torpid bowels; hard and lumpy motions; headache, drowsiness, dizziness; retention of urine.

Plumbum—Obstinate cases; dark motions, consisting of *small balls.*

Podophyllum—Pale or clay-coloured evacuations, mottled with green; Constipation following Diarrhoea; *Prolapsus ani;* sallow skin; restless sleep.

Sulphur—Painful distention of the abdomen; *habitual costivenes.*

Accessory Means—The diet in infants should be regulated according to directions on pages 20-23. Olive-oil and manna are often useful for infants—also malt extract and refined liquid paraffin. These may also be given to older children. By these last fresh vegetables—cabbage, turnips, onions—ripe fruit, oatmeal-porridge with treacle, and brown bread may be taken freely. A draught of water, especially on rising and retiring, is also advisable. Frictions with the warm hand or with *olive-oil* over the back and abdomen are often effectual in affording relief, and are applicable equally to infants and older children.

Children should early be habituated to solicit the action of the bowels every morning with regularity. Purgatives are to be strictly avoided. Regular exercise should be taken—also exercises designed to strengthen the abdominal muscles.

JAUNDICE (Icterus)

Definition—A disease due to derangement of the liver characterized by yellowness of many of the tissues of the body, especially the white-of-the eyes and finger-nails.

Symptoms—Yellow tinge, first of the white-of-the-eyes, then of the roots of the nails, next the face and neck, and finally the trunk and extremities. The urine becomes a deep orange or even mahogany colour, and stains the linen; the faeces pale yellow; there is Constipation or Diarrhoea; lassitude; anxiety; discomfort in liver region; bitter taste; and moderate fever. Often the bowels and relaxed from the food not being properly digested and occasioning irritation. There are also, usually depression of spirits, prostration of strength, and slowness of the pulse.

Causes—Chill, exposure, errors of diet, and emotional storms. (*Icterus neonatorum* or "jaundice of the newly-born" is not uncommon, coming on about the second or third day and lasting a few days. Its cause is not certain, and it is hardly to be considered a disease.)

Treatment—In a large number of cases, *Mercurius* will meet every requirement, and unless some other medicine is very clearly indicated it should be given every three hours.

Indications for the several Remedies

Aconitum—Jaundice from fright or cold; *febrile heat;* much pain below the ribs.

Chamomilla—Jaundice caused by *fits of passion.*

China—From indigestible substances, over-exertion, cold, when the disease assumes an intermittent character and when large doses of mercury have been given.

Mercurius Sol. 3x—One of the most useful medicines, when the patient has not been subjected to mercury under allopathic treatment.

Nux Vomica—Pain in the region of the liver; *Costiveness;* sickness.

Chronic cases may require *Chelid., Dig., Hydras., Nit.-Ac. Phos.,* or *Podoph.*

Accessory Means—Flannels wrung out of hot water, applied to the region of the liver, are good. Daily out-of-door exercise, regulation of the diet, and protection from atmospheric changes, are excellent *preventive.*

Chapter VII
DISEASES OF THE CUTANEOUS SYSTEM

STROPHULUS (Teething Rash)

Definition—A rash characterized by red papules (red strophulus) or white papules (white strophulus), round, of the size of a pin's head or millet-seed, and very itchy, which appears first on the body, afterwards on the face and limbs.

Causes—It is found only in infants and children, and is due to digestive disturbance and overclothing, and is often asociated with the first Dentition.

Indication for Treatment

Ant.-Curd.—Associated with Indigestion; white tongue, Vomiting, etc.

Calc.-Carb.—With chronic acidity; delicate children.

Chamomilla—This is generally the most efficatious remedy.

Puls.—Indigestion, tedency to Diarrhoea.

Accessory Means—An exclusive diet of milk; abundance of fresh air; moderate clothing; dusting the affected parts with a mixture of zinc oxide and strach powder.

ECZEMA

Definition—Eczema is a dermatitis (inflamation of the skin) which shows "the successive phases of Erythema, vesication, and an exudution which dries into scabs and which stiffens linen fabrics" (Granham Little).

Eczema is one of the most common of skin affections, and lasts a varying time according to the constitution of the patient, the treatment adopted, and other conditions.

No traces ramain after its disappearance.

Symptoms—In very young children it commences as an acute attack, which is prone to subside into a chronic form and as such to persist for a long time. The patient is usually rosy, healthy-looking, plump—perhaps if anything over-fat— of fine, fair complexion. Locally, we have redness; vesicles from which serous fluid oozes copiously and dries into yellowish scabs and crusts; itching; heat. Later, especially if the site of Eczema is scratched, pus-producing germs get in and cause pustules which form greenish-yellow scabs. In children Eczema typically and chiefly manifests itself on the *face* and *head*, starting usually below the eyes and spreading downwards over the face and upwards over the scalp.

Causes—Eczema within the definition given above may be due to any one of a large number of irritants: *mechanical* (such as are due to the friction caused by working a machine, riding a bicycle, or the irritation of woolen clothing); *chemical* (such as is due to the irritation of sugary urine in Diabetes or of faeces in the so-called "napkin-rash" of infants); *occupational* (such as is due to handling paints, petrol, antiseptics, photographic materials, shavings of certain woods, hair-dyes, soaps, etc.); *parasitic* (such as is due to the irritation of lice, itch-mites, etc.); but the Eczema of children described above, though it may be precipitated by exposure to cold or, less often, to heat, is an affection *from within*, an expression of a constitutional and hereditary predisposition, and might fairly be called "idiopathic"—hence at once (*a*) the necessity for "constitutional" treatment, and (*b*) the danger of strong outward applications which may "drive the trouble in." It is remarkable in this connexion that Eczema often alternates in the same individual or in members of the same family with such a constitutional disease as spasmodic Asthma.

Indications for Treatment

Ant.-Tart.—For *Eczema impetiginodes;* vesicles surrounded with red areola, especially about the nose, eyes, ears, neck, and shoulders.

Arsenicum—Burning, corrosive discharge from skin. In chronic cases it is of the greatest use.

Calc.-Carb.—Thick scales, with pus underneath; stools chalky; nutrition defective.

Croton Tig.—Severe itching, with sickness, or painful Diarrhoea.

Hepar.-Sulph.—In chronic cases.

Mercur.-Sol.—Bright-red, shining eruption, burning pain, brownish scabs, swollen glands.

Rhus Tox.—Much itching, worse at night. The most useful medicine for simple acute Eczema.

Sulphur—When situated chiefly on the head or vulva; violent itching; during convalescence.

Accesories—Crusts and scrabs should be softened by means of compresses of warm olive-oil and gently detached.

Serious or purulent fluid should never be allowed to accumulate under cakes of dried secretion. When the head is affected, the hair must be cut short.

A lotion of *Ant.-Tart.*, *Ars.*, or *Croion Tig.* may be used topically when the same remedy is being used internally. Ten grains of Trit. *Ant.-Tart.* 1x ten drops of Tinct. *Arsen.* 2x, or twenty drops of Tinct. *Croton Tig.* 1x may be added to eight ounces of distilled water, and used once or twice a day, or twenty drops of *Ol. Croton Tig.* mixed with an ounce of olive-oil may be employed instead of *Croton lotion.* When the irritation is excessive the following ointment will be of great utility: Nitrate of Bismuth, grs. 30; Lard, one ounce: mix. When the Eczema ceases to weep and reaches the scaly stage, a dry powder (such as plain starch powder or an ordinary dusting powder, composed of zinc oxide, boracic acid, and starch powder) may be used. Or an ointment may be used, such as plain lanolin or calendula ointment. The face must be protected from cold wind and hot sun, and must not be washed with soap. Oatmeal-water or tar-water may be used.

In acute Eczema involving large areas it is often good to put the child on an exculsive diet or milk or whey or rice and water for a few days, keeping the patient in bed at the same time.

In the more chronic Eczema the practice of drinking considerable quantities of plain water should be encouraged.

IMPETIGO (Contagiosa)

Impetigo, a common disease of infants, is a severe, contagious, purulent inflammation of the skin, with heat, or itching, and has been described as *Pustular Eczema* by some writers. It is characterized by an eruption of pustules grouped in clusters, having a tedency to run together, forming

irregularly-shaped, thick, moist, yellowish scabs or incrusta-
tions; and attacking the ear, nose, scalp, an face. No scars are
left after healing.

Causes—Inoculation with pus-producing germs. It
spreads rapidly in school from child to child.

Treatment—The scabs should be softened with warm
olive-oil and carefully bathed off; each raw spot should then
be touched with a weak mercurial ointment (*Ung. Hydrarg.
Nit. Dil.*). This should be done daily. Internally, *Hepar Sulph.* or
Viola Tric. should be given.

URICARIA (Nettle-rash)

Definition—An eruption of round or oval wheals, pale in
the centre, and red at the circumference, attended with
smarting and excessive itching, as though the parts had been
stung by nettles—hence the popular name.

Symptoms—Towards evening, or when getting warm in
bed, the patient feels an intolerable itching on the neck, arms,
or body, and on scratching soon discovers large *wheals* (the
eruption rapidly enlarging under the irritation of scratching)
which burn, tingle, or smart, and prove the source of great
discomfort.

Causes—The acute form as seen in children, is often due
to Indigestion or eating particular articels of food, as bitter
almonds, shell-fish, oatmeal, etc. It may also perhaps be
induced by a chill, or changes in the weather. Often there
seems no cause for it.

Indications for Treatment

Aconitum—When caused by a chill, or accompanied with
fever symptoms.

Antimonium Crud.—When caused by shell-fish, or almonds.

Apis Mell.—Sensations of stinging, burning, and prickling.

Dulcamara—Cases occurring in *damp* weather; much irritation.

Pulsatilla—When caused by fat, pastry, or pork.

Rhus Tox.—Small spots resembling flea-bites, with purplish swellings and intense irritation, particularly on the joints. It may also be used locally, replacing the *Veratrum V.* of the prescription below by *Rhus φ.*

Sulphur—Chronic Urticaria. Coming on when warm in bed.

Veratrum Viride—Intense pain and tingling. In the following preparation it may be used locally with great benefit:-

> B.   *Ver.-Viride φ*, gtts xx.
> Aqua,
> Spiritus V. R. } ā ā ℥ss.
> M.

Accessories—Remove the dietetic or other cause if there be one. Hot soda baths are often useful; so also is tar lotion.

INTERTRIGO—CHAFING—SORENESS OF INFANTS

Definition—Redness and chafing produced by the friction of two folds of skin, especially in fat children. It is seen in the groin, armpits, and neck. Sometimes a fluid is exuded, the acridity of which increases the local mischief, and an offensive raw surface is soon produced.

Intertrigo differs from Eczema in its acute course, and in the character of the secretion, which is clear, and does not stiffen linen. When confined to the buttocks and perineum, it may be difficult to distinguish from the rash of congenital Syphilis.

Indications for Treatment

Calc.-Carb.—In scrofulous children.

Cham.—Very efficacious in infants.

Lycopodium—In very obstinate cases.

Mercurius Sol.—Rawness and great soreness.

Sulphur—In chronic cases ; much itching.

Accessories—The parts should be well washed with cold or tepid water, and carefully dried, two or three times a day; a piece of linen, saturated with *Calendula lotion* (a teaspoonful of the tincture to a tumbler of water), may be laid between the opposing surfaces; or, in bad cases, a lotion, composed of one part of *Tincture of Hydrastis* to five parts of *Glycerine* and five parts of water, may be applied in the same manner; dusting the chafed parts with a fine powder consisting of equal parts of *Lycopodium* and *Oxide of Zinc*, or of Fuller's earth, is also useful.

CHILBLAINS (Pernio) AND CHAPS

Definition—"A localized Erythema attended with exudation, occurring . . . in certain predisposed persons in cold and damp weather" (Sequeira). It commonly affects the fingers and toes, but also the ears and nose.

Causes—Chilblains generally occur in frosty weather from exposure to a low temperature, sudden changes, damp, warming the feet at the fire when cold or damp. The inflamation chiefly affects children and young people.

Indications for Treatment

Agaricus—Stinging pains in the swellings; also when ulcerated.

Arnica—Hard, shining, painful, and itching swellings; in the early stage.

Petrol—Broken, itching, burning chilblains.

Pulsatilla—Livid redness, itching and heating in the swelling, and worse towards evening.

Rhus Tox.—When the parts are much inflamed, or blistered.

Accessories—All the remedies may be used externally as well as internally, in the form of lotion or cerate except Arnica, which should never be used for *broken* chillblains. *Glycerine*, *Glycerine-of-starch*, or one part of *Glycerine* mixed with two parts of *Eau-de-Colonge*, is an excellent remedy for Chilblains, Chapped-hands, *fissures* or *cracks*. It removes the stinging, burning sensations and makes the parts soft and supple. Ulcerated Chilblains may require a poultice, or other mild application, until relieved. *Aconite*, mother tincture, may be rubbed on unbroken Chilblains, or they may be painted with *Tincture of Iodine*.

Extremes of temperature are to be avoided, especially cold stone floors, suddenly approaching the fire after coming in from the cold, warming the feet on the fender, or the hands close to the fire. Warm gloves, thick socks or stockings, thick boots should be worn. The hands should be dipped into cold water and then subjected to prolonged friction with a warm dry towel.

As Chilblains generally occur in children whose circulation is defective, plenty of exercise in the open air, the free use of the skipping-rope, and wholesome nutritious diet including a fair amount of fat, are necessary to prevent their recurrence. Pork, veal, salted meats, and irritating, indigestible kinds of food, are inadmissible.

PARASITIC DISEASES OF THE SKIN
(Morbi cutis Parasitici)

The parasitic diseases most commonly found among children are the following:-

Tinea Tonsurans—This affection, known as the common *scrufy ringworm*, occurs most frequently in strumous children. Being contagious it is not neccessarily associated with deranged general health. It occurs mostly between the second and twelfth years, as irregularly circular patches, varying in size from that of a sixpence to that of a penny piece, the hairs of which look withered, dry, thickened, and as if cut off at a short distance from the roots. The skin is red or scaly.

Treatment—The quickest and most certain treatment of ringworms of the scalp is the X-rays. If these are not available the daily inunction of *Chrysarobin ointment* should be tried. This, it should be remembered, stains linen, and, more important, if it touches the eyes, causes an acute Conjunctivitis. To know if the treatment has been successful, the application should be stopped for a month and a careful watch instituted to see whether any small scaly patches or stumps appear (Whitfield).

Pityriasis Versicolor—This commences as small reddish points, with irritation and itching inreased by warmth, and followed by irregular, fawn-coloured patches, dry, rough, scaly at the edge, and slightly elevated, and from which scurf can be detached by rubbing. The patches vary in size from half an inch to three or four inches in diameter, and occur mostly where the body is in *contact with flannel*, particularly on the chest, neck, and abdomen. Like the preceding, it is contagious, and its spread is favoured by uncleanly habits. It is also called *Chloasma*. It is specially common in tuberculous subjects.

The treatment consists in the diligent use of a 3% *Salicylic acid ointment*.

Scabies—Itch—This disease is caused by the presence of a minute animal parasite, the *Acarus scabiei*, which burrows under the skin, and gives rise to an eruption and an intolerable itching. The eruption is vesicular, presenting numerous small watery conical pimples, and appears most frequently between the fingers, and the bend of the arm in children, or on the thighs and buttocks and lower part of the abdomen in infants, by whom it is occasionally contracted from uncleanly servants or nurses. The irritation increases at night and in bed.

Treatment—Sulphur is the great enemy to parasitic life, and its local application is the most effective means of destroying the *Acarus*. After thoroughly rubbing the whole body with soft-soap and warm water, then washing in a hot bath, or with hot water, and wiping thoroughly dry, the superficial and effete cuticle is removed, and the burrows and parasites freely exposed; the ointment should then be well rubbed in and allowed to remain on the body all night. On the following morning a tepid bath, using yellow soap, to wash off the ointment left on overnight, completes the cure. If the application of the ointment and the ablutions be not thorough, the process should be repeated once or twice. But *Sulphur ointment* must not be continued too long, or it will produce an irritable state of the skin, which may be taken for a persistence of the disease. All contaminated linen should be boiled in water; other garments should be well ironed with a hot iron, or exposed to hot air at a temperature of not less that 150° to 180° Fahr., or well fumigated with the vapour of *Sulphur*, to destroy any insects or ova concealed in the textures of the linen. The cure is often retarded, and the disease conveyed to others, by neglecting to carry out these suggestions thoroughly.

Sep. Calc.-Carb., and *Sulph.* are sometimes useful, administered interanally; *Sepia* in Ringworm, *sulphur* in Scabies, and

Calcarea in general unhealthy states of the skin, and for the debility which favours these diseases.

Pediculosis (Lousiness) — This disease is caused by the presence of animal parasites (*Pediculus capitis,* the comonest — *P. corporis, P. pubis*) and their eggs ("nits"). It is easily contracted through the careless use of hair-brushes, and is by no means confined to the poorer or dirtier classes. It creates intense itching which results in scratching; the scratches are apt to get infected with pus-producing germs and thus to become the seat of *Impetigo contagiosa.* An excellent preparation for killing *Pediculi capitis* is *Oil of Sassafras.* The oil is thoroughly soaked into the hair and left on all night under a bathing-cap. The elemination of the lice is expedited by cutting the hair short. The eggs or "nits" are tiny whitish bodies fastened to the hair-shafts by a glutinuous material. They are readily distinguished from the fine powder of scurf or dandruff by the fat that the latter is readily brushed off, but the nits stick. The nits are best removed by a small-toothed comb. Infected clothes should be "stoved" or destroyed.

STINGS AND BITES OF INSECTS

Internal Treatment

Aconitum — Swelling, inflamation, fever.

Arnica — After the subsidence of fever if there remain tenderness and smarting.

Ledum Palustre — Said to be a great efficacy in the mosquito bites.

Rhus Tox. — Has often been used with good effect.

Accessories — Washing blue or ammonia should be applied locally or the remedy given internally may be employed as a lotion externally as the same time. If the sting of the insect be left in the wound it should be extracted as soon as possible.

———————

Chapter VIII

MISCELLANEOUS AFFECTIONS

CRYING

Significance or Crying—The crying of an infant is expressive, and varies much in character. "In cerebral affections it is sharp, short, and sudden. In lesions of the abdomen, exciting pain, it is prolonged. In inherited Syphilis, it is high-pitched and hoarse. In inflammatory diseases of the larynx, it is hoarse, and may be whispering. In inflammatory diseases of the chest, and in severe Rickets, the child is usually quiet and unwilling to cry, on account of the action interfering with the respiratory functions" (*Dr. Eustace Smith*).

Causes—In many instances, infantile crying and fretfulness depends upon some mechanical cause—tight or creased clothing, wet napkins, the prick or scratch of pin, improper or excessive feeding, etc. Crying is also the language by which its wants are expressed; but it is a mistake to suppose that the child should be presented to the breast, or that it is hungry merely because it cries. The time that has elapsed since the previous nursing will determine the necessity or otherwise for feeding the child. Water may be all that it requires, and it should have this freely. Crying is, however, often due to *Colic*, wind, or other symptoms of Indigestion in hand-fed children, or in infants suckeled by unsuitable wet-nurses. For a proper investigation of the cause of crying, the infant should be fully undressed in a room of comfortable temperature. By this method the form and movements of the chest and abdomen; the state of the skin, whether hot or cool, moist or dry; the presence or absence of any eruption, and any other peculiarity present, may then be easily detected.

Indications for Treatment

Aconitum—Hot, dry skin; full pulse; restlessness.

Belladonna—Crying without apparent cause; heat of the head; sparkling eyes; flushed cheeks; starting during sleep; Constipation.

Bryonia—Constipation.

Camphor—After *Chamomilla* when *Cham.* proves insufficient, and the child seems in great pain.(Dose: One or two drops upon a little loaf sugar; after crushing it well, small portion of the powder may be placed on the tongue.)

Chamomilla—Constant crying, with *drawing up of the legs;* pain in, or distention of, the abdomen; looseness of the bowels.

Coffea—Nervousness, restlessness, and tossing about; sleeplessness.

Accessories—Hot flannel applied to the abdomen, or rubbing with the warmed hand; placing the child on the knee with the stomach downwards, and patting the back gently, will often prove soothing. A warm bath, as described on page 15, is sometimes very beneficial.

MORBUS COXAE—TUBERCULOUS DISEASE OF THE HIP-JOINT

Definition—Tuberculous inflamation, sometimes originating in the synovial membrane (the membrane which covers the joints, secreting the "synovial" fluid which lubricates the joints and tendons), and sometimes in the articulating surfaces of the bones, commonly met with in children, and before the disease assumes an aggressive form, often attributed to "growing-pains."

Symptoms—The first distinctive symptoms are—slight limping pain in walking, with disinclination to allow the entire weight of the body to rest on the affected limb. At this state, the pain is *chiefly referred to the knee.* There may be even slight swelling in the knee-point, so as to lead to error regarding the real nature of the disease. This is probably due to pressure on, or irritation of, the branch of the obturator nerve, distributed to the capsular ligament, and *ligamenum teres,* referred to the terminal cutaneous branches of the same nerve. The real seat of the pain may be proved by pressing either the front or back of the hip-joint, or by jerking the thigh-bone against the joint, as by a sharp tap on the heel, when pain will be felt in the hip. On close observation, the limb will probably be found slightly flexed, and there may be feverishness and restlessness in the evening, and perhaps slight twitching of the thigh in the night. As the disease progresses, the lameness becomes very decided, and the nates of the affected side waste and become flabby; the limb is shortened, either by caries of the neck of the femur, or by ulceration and destruction of the ligaments of the joint, and consequent dilocation of the joint upwards on the *dorsum ilii.* This is termed *spontaneous dislocation.* There is increased fullness about the limb, the pains increase in severity, especially at night, and there are often violent startings of the

limb during sleep. Abscesses form and afterwards burst on
the nates (buttocks) or groin, or burrow deeply and discharge
their contents into the rectum. *Wasting of the nates* of the
affected side is one of the earliest symptoms of the disease of
hip.

The *duration* of the disease varies from two to three
months to several years. But it is much modified, both as to
duration and results, by skilful treatment.

Indications for Treatment

Aconitum—If recognized in its early stages, a few doses of
Acon. may be of service; the presence of fever further indicates
this medicine.

Belladonna—In the early stage when the patient suffers
great pain.

Calcarea Carb.—At the commencement of the second stage,
when suppuration is threatening.

Colocynth—Useful when there is much neuralgic pain
attending the disease.

Mercurius Cor.—When the patient has a sallow complexion;
syphilitic taint.

Silica—When ulceration has taken place in the bones.

Sulphur—As an intercurrent remedy in protected cases.

Additional Remedies—*Ars., Cantharis, China, Graph., Hep.-
S., Nit.-Ac., Phosph., Puls., Rhus Tox., Staph.*

Accessory Means—Rest, with the limb kept straight, and
absence of the articular pressure; the latter is probably the
more important element; surgical appliances are necessary to
ensure it. The diet should be nourishing and include *Cod-liver
oil.* Pure air, especially change to the seaside, will expedite the
cure. When abscesses discharge, they should be kept free
from foetor by means of *Carbolic oil.*

LATERAL CURVATURE OF THE SPINE—SKOLIOSIS
(Gr., σκολιός, crooked)

Definition—A deviation of the spine to one side or other of the middle line.

Causation—Such curvature may be due to Rickets, in which case together with muscular weakness there is softening of the bones and other supporting structure. Or to Infantile Paralysis, or to Tuberculous Disease of the Spine. But by Scoliosis, not otherwise qualified, we mean *static* or *adolescent* Scoliosis, a condition due to diminished muscular tone. Where Scoliosis becomes habitual, there is in addition rotation of the vertebrae (usually the dorsal), and this leads to deformity of the whole throax, the front of the chest being conspicuously flattened on one side and pushed forward on the other. The hips and scapulae are observed to be quite asymmetrical.

Age and Type of Patients—The following excellent description of a typial case in a girl of twelve is quoted from Fairbank: "She is a pale, thin, unhealthy-looking child with an adenoid facies. She has stooped for some years; her chest is flat, and the respiratory movements are feeble. Many of her teeth are carious; her tonsils are enlarged and spetic; adenoids are present; she has chronic enlargement of the cervical glands, below and behind the angles of the jaw, proving the absorption of septic meaterial from the mouth and throat. She is anaemic, and a haemic murmur may be heard over the praecordium. Her school hours are too long; when in school she sits on a form, and when writing is allowed to assume any position her tired muscles suggest; the schoolroom is badly ventilated. Her play-horus she usually spends indoors. When standing she usually keeps one knee flexed and the pelvis tilted down on the same side; there is knock-knee, more marked on one side; both feet are 'weak.' Her mother gives a history of snoring at night and of frequent colds and sore throats; the child never sleeps with the windows open on this accounts. Constipation is troublesome."

Treatment—The typical case just quoted indicates the general lines along which treatment should be instituted. The general health must be attended to and the patient placed under the best hygienic conditions. Bad teeth, septic tonsils, and adenoids should be removed. She should be trained in breathing exercises. School hours may need to be shortened. An open-air life must be encouraged, open-air exercise being graduated according to her strength. She must not be allowed to stand too long at a time, and the "standing at ease" position should be discouraged. "A scoliotic patient should always use a chair, not a stool or form, and the back should have a cushion or pad adjusted so as to fit into the lumbar concavity. The desk should be sloping be close to the chair, and a footstool should be fixed beneath it" (Fairbank). In addition the patient should be massaged, and Ling's Swedish exercises from a person specially qualified to give them. The question whether and at what stage a patient will require a mechaincal support should be referred to an orthopaedic specialist. The tendency to-day is to do without these things, and to depend upon physical exercise and general hygiene.

SWELLING OF INFANTS' BREASTS

The breasts of infants usually contain at birth a secretion resembling milk. This, if uninterfered with, is soon absorbed, and the swellings subside. But many nurses will not leave nature to have her own way; they consider it necessary to effect a speedy remove of the fluid by sqeezing the breasts, or else to rupture the "nipple-strings." This may shortly lead to inflammation (*Mastitis*) and even Mammary Abscess. At a later date it may produce retracted nipples, a disfigurement and a handicap to women. Apart from any ill-usage, inflammation of the breasts is quite common in the second week, and may go on to suppuration.

Indications for Treatment

Aconitum—If the inflamation is high.
Arnica—If the redness is but slight.
Belladonna—If the redness assume an erysipelatous character.
Hepar. S.—If suppuration has taken place.
The medicine chosen should be given every four hours.

RUPTURED NAVEL (Umbilical Hernia)

Definition—A protrusion from the abdominal cavity through the navel-ring, where it forms a smooth, ovoid, tense tumour, easily returnable by pressure. It is sometimes congenital, but more frequently occurs soon after the separation of the navel cord.

Causes—Violent crying or straining of the infant while the integuments which close the umbilical ring are but imperfectly developed.

Treatment—Should there be any signs of a protrusion at birth, or soon after, a circular piece of cork should be applied, somewhat convex on both sides covered with soft leather, and secured by a moderately tight-fitting bandage around the abdomen. A flat piece of sheet lead, or ivory, protected with soft leather, with the convex surface over the aperture, may be substituted for the cork. If the pad slips off the part, it should be secured by cross pieces of adhesive plaster. If the pad is nicely applied, and continued for one or two months, a radical cure may be expected.

Remedies—*Nux Vomica* at night, and *Sulphur* in the morning, are recommended, and perhaps facilitate the cure.

INCONTINENCE OF URINE—WETTING THE BED

This is a frequent and troublesome affection of children, consisting of partial or complete loss of power to retain the urine. From the age of three, at any rate, a child should have control of the bladder. The most comon form is *Enuresis nocturna*—wetting the bed; in rarer cases the child may have an almost incessant urging to pass water, which, if not responded to, results in a painless, involuntary discharge. If the child be troubled with a cough, the inconvenience is much increased, as during each paroxysm the urine is apt to escape. The affection is most common in children three or four to fourteen or sixteen years of age, and is most frequent at night.

Causes—Apart from general diseases such as Diabetes, Rheumatism, Epilepsy, inflammation of the spinal cord, or mental deficiency, of which is may be but one manifestation, enuresis may be caused by (*a*) some lesion in the urinary tract, such as Calculus, Bacilluria or Cystitis (inflammation of the bladder); (*b*) abnormality of the urine itself, either excessive quantity (due to drinking too much fluid in the evening) or excessive acidity; (*c*) reflexly through the nervous system by thread-worms, Phimosis, adherent foreskin, adenoids, etc. ; (*d*) some inherent defect in the nervous control of the bladder.

Treatment—*Belladonna* and *Calc.-Carb.* are the most useful remedies. *Causticum* often acts well. Quarter-grain doses of *thyroid extract*, gradually increased, are useful where there is reason to believe that the thyroid secretion is deficient (dry harsh skin, dull expression, thick lips, chilliness, Constipation).

If there is no reason to suspect thyroid deficiency, and if *Bell.* (1 x or 3 x or higher), *Calc.-Carb.* and *Causticum* (in this order) have been tried (along with all accessory measures) without success, then a trial should be made of *Belladonna* in substantial doses, beginning with five drops of the mother tincture three times a day and rapidly increasing until fifteen to twenty drops are taken four times a day. If the enuresis stops under this dosage it should be continued for three or four weeks and then gradually diminished to the vanishing point.

Accessory Means—Tolle causam ("remove the casue") is obviously the first injunction to remember. If there is calculus or anything of a surgical nature, it must be surgically removed. If there is Bacilluria (see page 183), Thread-worms (page 155), Adenoids (page 131), they must be treated. Adenoids may have to be removed. Phimosis must be remedied by circumcision. Excessive acidity of the urine, not a common cause of Enuresis, may be remedied by giving alkalies such as bicarbonate of soda, but is probaly relieved equally well by giving the indicated homoeopathic remedy, as well as by limiting the starch in the diet. Fluid should be taken freely (e.g. plain water and bland drinks) in the early part of the day, but none after five o'clock. The mother or nurse should be quite certain that the child fully empties his bladder before getting into bed, as a child very tried or sleepy is apt to shirk this. If the child is found (as is often the case) to wet during his early sleep, he should be waken up after two hours or even after one hour, and later on again, when the parents retire to rest. A helpful adjunct to treatment is to raise the foot of the bed nine or twelve inches. The child should sleep on a hard mattress, with light clothing, and should not lie on his back; this may be prevented by fixing an empty cotton-reel so that on turning on his back the reel may press into the muscles. At bedtime an occasional warm bath at 90° to 98° Fahr., or a warm sitz bath, is often of great value in this disease, and greatly contributes to the success of the general treatment. Sponging the lower part of the back with hot water at bedtime is said to cure some cases of incontinence in children. Patients should take much open-air exercise, and have ablutions with *cold* water every morning: this with the subsequent drying should not occupy more than a few minutes.

Corporal punishment will work no cure. The fear of it increases the tendency to urinate in the case of nervous children. It should only be resorted to when incontinence is the result of an indolent habit of neglecting the natural desire.

BACILLURIA

Definition—An infection of the urniary tract with *Bacillus coli* (rarely with *Bacillus proteus*).

Symptoms—There may be *Bacilli coli*, even in fair abundance, in the urine, without any symptoms. But often there is slight fever, up to 100°, the child is out of sorts, languid and fretful; no urinary symptoms are complained of, but the water, which is acid, is cloudy and turbid, with a stale "ancient fish-like odour," and contains pus. If there is actual Cystitis (inflammation of the bladder), there will be great frequency and pain and scalding in passing water. During the course of a simple Bacilluria, there may be sudden exacerbation of symptoms, with sharp rise of temperature to 103° or 104° (accompanied perhaps by rigors or attack of collapse) with pain in the loin (nearly always the right loin). These attacks may come on quite suddenly when the child is in good health, and they are then apt to be very puzzling, because the child does not complain of any symptom that points to the urinary system. Examination of the urine shows the presence of pus and swarms (perhaps a pure culture) of colon bacilli, and a diagnosis is at once made of acute Pyelitis (inflammation of the pelvis of the kidney) due to *Bac. coli.*

Causes—The fact that girls are much more prone to this infection than boys are, suggests strongly that the colon bacilli migrate from the anus to the vulva and so trek up the urinary tract to the kidney. It is possible that intestinal worms (*Oxyurides*), which undoubtedly migrate to the female vulva, carry colon bacilli with them. Recent opinion inclines, however, strongly to the vies that the usual route of infection in cases at any rate of acute Pyelitis, is from the ascending colon to the right kidney, a belief favoured by the fact that there has usually been some intestinal disturbance and perhaps, as a consequence, some injury of the intestinal mucous membrane, before the onset of the Pyelitis. Some have believed that the appendix is the source of trouble and advocate removal of the appendix as part of the treatment.

Treatment—The disease is one that has only lately been recognized, and there are no records of its homoeopathic treatment. The disease, however, readily yields to the simple device of giving an alkali like citrate of potash, which may be combined with bicarbonate of soda, in quantities sufficient to make the urine alkaline. To effect this it may be necessary to give ten or fifteen grains three or four times a day even to infants. Older children will want more. Older children, too, in addition to receiving alkalies, should have milk cut out of their diet. An autogenous vaccine, that is a vaccine made from the patient's own bacilli, is quite often useful in improving the patient's general health. If there is any intestinal irregularity, this should be treated (pages 150-160).

GLOSSARY

Abscess A gathering, a collection of pus.

Agglutination Adhesion of two surfaces.

Alae Nasi The cartilaginous sides of the nose.

Anaemia Impoverished state of the blood.

Anus The orifice of the large bowel.

Arachnoid The smooth cobweb-like investment of the brain.

Areolar Tissue The tissue which connects the various component parts of the body.

Asthenic Want of strength.

Atrophy Wasting.

Cachexia A bad habit of body.

Caries Ulceration of bone or teeth.

Cartilage Gristle.

Casein The Nitrogenized principle of milk.

Cell-proliferation Cell-bearing.

Cellular Tissue Same as Areolar tissue.

Cerebral   Relating to the brain.

Chloasma   Liver spots.

Chyle   The milk-like fluid absorbed by the lacteal vessels digested food.

Cicatrices   Scars

Coma   Torpor; lethargic sleep.

Congenital   From birth.

Congestion   Undue fulness of the blood-vessels in an organ.

Conjunctiva   The lining membrane of the eyelids and the front part of the globes of the eye.

Convalescence   The state of recovery.

Cutaneous   Belonging to the skin.

Cuticle   The external layer of skin.

Defluction   Discharge of excessive secretions.

Depurating   Cleansing from impurities.

Desquamation   Scaling of the skin.

Diagnosis   The distinction of diseases.

Diathesis   Constitutional predisposition to disease.

Dorsum Ilii   The back of the hip bone.

Dysponoea   Dificult breathing.

Efflorescence   The Pulverescence of crystals by the removal of their moisture on exposure to the air.

Effluvia   Exhalation from putrefying substances.

Effusion   The pouring out of fluid.

Emaciation Wasting.

Emphysema Infiltration of air into areolar tissues of the lungs or the dilation of the air-cells.

Ephemeral Of short duration.

Epithelial Scales The superficial scales of mucous membrane.

Epithelium The superficial layer of mucous membrane.

Erosion Destruction by ulceration.

Eustachian Tubes The canal connecting the ear with the throat.

Exanthemata Eruptive fevers.

Excoriation Abrasion of the skin.

Faridization Applying fardic or induced electricity.

Febricula Simple fever.

Femur The thigh bone.

Fibro-cartilage A substance intermediate between cartilage and ligament, which constitutes the base of the ears, the rings of the windpipe, etc.

Fluctuation The undulations of fluid in the cavity.

Fontanelles The cartilaginous spaces in the head of an infant at the juncture of the bones.

Gangrene Mortification.

Gastric Pertaining to the stomach.

Gonorrhoea A contagious discharge from the urinary organs.

Haematuria Passing blood with the urine.

Haemorrhage Loss of blood.

Heartburn A hot sensation in pit of stomach.

Homogeneous Consisting of similar elements.

Hygienic Relating to the preservation of health.

Ileum The lower three-fifths of the small bowels.

Incubation The time between the reception of a poison and the occurrence of its action.

Innervation The functions of the nervous system.

Insomnia Restlessness in sleep.

Lachrymation A profuse secretion of tears.

Lactation The process of secreting and supplying milk, of nursing, or suckling.

Larynx The upper part of the air passage.

Leptothrix Buccalis A parasitic plant.

Lesion An injury or disease of some organ or tissue.

Leucorrhoea Whites.

Ligamentum teres The round ligament connecting the thigh and hip bones.

Lymph The fluid in the lymphatic vessels.

Mammae Breasts.

Meatus The ear canal.

Membrana Tympani The drum of the ear.

Mesenteric Glands The lymphatic glands of the small intestine.

Metastasis The removing from one part to another.

Miasm Contagious effluvia.

Molars The double or grinding teeth.

Mucous Membrane The lining membrane of the digestive organs.

Nates The buttocks.

Nidus A nest.

Oedema Local dropsy of cellular tissue.

Orbicularis Palpebrarum A small muscle which close and protects the eye.

Otorrhoea Discharge from the ear.

Ozaena Foetid discharge from the nose.

Pabulum Food, or means of subsistence. Usually spoken of in regard to the germ theory of contagion. Those who are susceptible to a disease are said to afford "pabulum" for the disease germ to subsist upon the multiply. The phrase "a suitable soil" is sometimes used instead.

Parotitis Mumps.

Pathologial Characteristic of disease.

Pedunculated Having a peduncle or stalk.

Pericarditis Inflamation of the sac which surrounds the heart.

Peritonitis Inflammation of the lining of the abdominal cavity.

Pertussis Whooping-cough.

Ptyalism Salivation; increased flow of saliva.

Phymosis Swelling of the foreskin.

Pneumo-gastric Nerve The eighth pair of nerves, distributed to the lungs and stomach.

Pneumatic Aspirator An instrument for drawing out fluids from closed cavities. It consists of a hollow needle which is thrust into the cavity, the needle being attached to an air pump, the action of which draws out the fluid.

Prophylactic   Preventive.

Purulent   Of the character of pus.

Psychical   Relating to the mental and moral faculties.

Rales   A whistling, cooing, or rattle in the chest.

Rectum   Terminal part of the bowel.

Regimen   Rule of diet.

Resolution   The subsidence of inflammation without suppuration, etc; the dispersion of swellings.

Rima Glottidis   The aperture of the windpipe.

Roseola   Scarlet red.

Rubeola   Measles.

Salivation   See Ptyalism.

Secretion   Fluid separated from the blood.

Sensorium   The centre of perception in the brain.

Sequeale   Secondary disease following another.

Serum   The watery portion of the blood.

Sloughing   The mortifying or dying of the tissues.

Sordes   Accumualtion of dried and discoloured mucus on the teeth.

Sporules and Spores   The reproductive parts of seeds.

Sputa   The spittle, or expectoration.

Stamina   Inherent force or vitality.

Stasis   Standing, stagnation.

Struma Scrofula.

Styptic An astringent.

Suppuration Formation of pus.

Sutures The junction of the bones of the skull.

Syncope Fainting.

Synovial Membrane A membrane attached to tendons and lining joints, and secreting a kind of lubricating oil—the synovial fluid.

Syphilis A venereal poison.

Tabes Mesenterica Consumption of the bowels.

Tenesmus Straining of the bowels after a motion.

Trachea The lower part of the windpipe.

Tubercle The early deposit in the organs of scrofulous and consumptive persons.

Tuberculosis The morbid state that gives rise to tubercles.

Tubular Fibrils Minute or ultimate fibres.

Turgescence Swelling from excess of fluid.

Tympanitic Distended like a drum.

Tympanum The drum of the ear.

Ulcers Open sores.

Uvula The pendulous body which hangs from the middle of the soft palate.

Variola Smallpox.

Vascular Abounding in blood-vessels.

Vertebrae The spine bones.

Vesicles Pimples containing fluid.

Vesicular Having the appearance of vesicles.

Virus Poison

Vulva The external female genitals.

Zymotic (Leaven) Contagious diseases.

THERAPEUTIC INDEX